Shared Heartbeats

Shared Heartbeats

Navigate Endometriosis and IVF with Knowledge, Perseverance, and Self-Love

Annika Östberg

Contents

Dedication

This book is dedicated with love and light to all women who suffer from endometriosis and have challenges getting pregnant. May you find peace in your heart, ease in your days and become free from pain. May you release yourself from harsh judgments while finding yourself in my story.

This book is also dedicated to those in my life who have been my greatest guides, people from all walks of my life, spirits, Source, and most importantly, my twins. They were the greatest fighters in my belly, as there were several times that we thought we lost them. They continue to be the greatest fighters who teach me a lot about life and continue to support me every day.

Once again, I need to dedicate this book to my precious miracle twins, Emilia, and Emil! She is wise, my warrior daughter who reminds me to be in the present moment, to enjoy daily life, and to have fun. Emil is my heartful soul-son who always shares his heartful love in the most beautiful ways. He brings me such joy and lifts me up.

And to my partner in crime, my husband Magnus, who still adores me and lets me know that often! He has been my rock, the love of my life, who inspires me to new adventures and encourages me to follow my heart.

The three of you are the sun in my life, the moon to my nights, and the deep joy in my heart. I look forward to the many more life adventures we will experience together as we continue this life. Thank you from the bottom of my heart for always caring for me. I Love you.

Foreword
Liselott Schönberg

In the rhythm of life, we often stumble upon stories that echo the universal song of resilience. "Shared Heartbeats" is one such melody woven with the threads of my dearest friend's journey—a journey that transformed her into a warrior, a beacon of strength, and an unwavering force against life's uncertainties.

"Shared Heartbeats" is not just a story; it's a guide—a guide for those facing similar storms, offering insights into endometriosis, infertility, and the emotional rollercoaster of IVF. Beyond the medical intricacies, Annika, with her profound knowledge, emphasizes the significance of practicing self-love and mindfulness and how alternative treatments and medicine can lend support. It sheds light on the importance of knowledge—knowledge that empowers, heals, and paves the way for informed decisions.

Having had the privilege of working in a company dedicated to supporting IVF clinics, I am acutely aware of the profound impact that endometriosis can have on fertility. The intricate dance of science and emotion involved in the in vitro fertilization process made me even more attuned to the challenges that

Annika faced, and equally made me more deeply impressed by the resilience with which she navigated through them.

As you journey through these pages, may you find not only comfort, understanding, and knowledge but also inspiration and a companion in Annika's wealth of experience.

With love,

Liselott Schönberg

A dear friend of Annika's

Opening

"May you be proud of the work you do, the person you are, and the difference you make."

— Abigail Johnson

There I was, sitting in an overcrowded room with a lot of people, trying to avoid staring at the women with baby bellies. It was a birthday party, and the two topics being discussed were: pregnancy and soccer. I don't like soccer and pregnancy doesn't like me, unfortunately. As usual, I try to look interested in my friend's conversations. Then it hits me, this time hard. What is this crap anyway? Why am I even sitting here? I don't want to listen to any of this. I am really trying to survive another party where most of my friends are expecting. The women are talking about everything related to being pregnant while the men are focused on soccer. It makes me want to throw up. I feel left out, full of shame and sad. I am not one of them. I don't fit in, again. I just want to go home. I want to be at home. I don't want to be here pretending to be all right when in reality, everything is wrong.

What makes things worse is when I see all the sad eyes peering over at me. I can actually feel them too. They don't know what to say to me either. They've forgotten how to converse with me as a friend. When they hear that I am still struggling with horrible, heavy bleedings. They become speechless. I hate when they feel sorry for me. I don't want their sorrow or pity. It sucks, but it's all I have ever known and nothing seems to be changing for the better.

If you picked this book up, I suspect that some of these feelings and experiences belong to you as well. Maybe you are tired of people feeling sorry for you. Perhaps too many family members and friends seem to keep asking if you are feeling better, if you've found a way to get pregnant yet, if your bleedings have subsided or if your debilitating cramps have gotten better. Maybe they wonder too, if you have gotten any help. You tell yourself that they just have your best interest in mind, that they want you to be alright, but it is hard for them to hear that it is still the same. Maybe your friends and family have gotten like my friends did where they may not know what to say anymore.

Women like us continue to experience a tsunami of feelings, over and over again, with surges filled with ebb and flows. There are so many personal struggles that develop when we go for years in this mode. It becomes overwhelming and exhausting. Life feels rough, without a lot of joy and soon you can feel so lost with nowhere to turn to. Then, you discover my book. Perhaps by divine chance. Perhaps through a recommendation. You now have a place to turn to. This book is trusting support, guidance, understandings, tools, and ideas. This book can become your dedicated companion. That is why I wrote it.

I wish, from the bottom of my heart, that sharing my story with you can give you much-needed support, information, preparation, courage, joy, and even some laughs during your unique journey. This book is a trusted and dedicated friend to read and talk to. If you are a partner or a friend to someone going through these womanly challenges, you can support them by reading this book. You will better understand endometriosis, trouble with getting pregnant and the IVF process. You will also learn or get new ideas about the thoughts and feelings experienced when going on this this type of journey. You will learn how to take care of yourself and support yourself, your partner and honor your beautiful body.

I believe life is a journey, and we experience things to grow, learn and evolve. When I was in the middle of heavy bleedings and all the different treatments, I struggled a lot with finding purpose and meaning with life. I went further and further spiraling down the black deep hole of depression. But I quickly learned that we are so much stronger than we think. I was recently listening to a song by Swedish DJ and record producer Aviccii. The lyrics went, *"Wake me up when it's all over."* That was how I felt many times. *"Let me sleep like a bear and wake up to a lovely spring when the sunlight comes through the light green leaves on the trees, and everything is cozy warm and smells great! And it is all over."*

He continues with, *"When I'm wiser and I'm older."* That sounded great too, resonating deep into my soul, like God sent a solution: just skip this hard part of my life and continue later when it's okay again and only if I really want to. Soon, I will be on the other side of it all. But, if all the struggles and pain could just disappear, I would not be the same person as I am today: a person that has gained so much wisdom and joy in one body. Also, a person that made it through the dark side many times, came out on the other side and finally made it all the way out to write this book. I am now the version of myself who can help support women struggling with heavy bleedings, endometriosis, cysts, or IVF right now.

This is a book filled with a lot of personal experience,

wisdom, tools and hope to make your life easier, more enjoyable, better, and happier. I want to remind you too, that we all are so much stronger than we think, so much more beautiful, smarter, and confident enough to grasp the importance of following your heart. We just need a reminder now and then. Your life is happening for you, not against you. This book will help you to get in a healthier mindset, give you support tools, and ways to walk more smoothly through this phase of your life with the ups and downs.

Here is a fun, lighter and favorite quote I adore:

"Strong women never give up.
We might need a coffee, a cry, or a day in bed, but we always come back stronger."
Author unknown.

I am strong. I also never forget that I am a **Warrior Queen**. I have fallen so many times and the hurt has been on the level of unbearable many times. I wanted to give up, but I always picked up my pieces, put myself back together again and rose back up. I became taller, prouder, stronger, and more grateful. I continue to work hard to choose positive thoughts and feelings because I WANT life to be beautiful, fun, healthy and wonderful.

What do you choose? I would be happy to hear any thoughts, insights, or anything that you experience during your journey and by reading this book.

May Light, Love and Laughter be your guides.

Annika ~

Chapter 1
The Warrior Within

"When we assert intuition, we are therefore like the starry night: we gaze at the world through a thousand eyes."

— *Clarissa Pinkola Estés, PHD*

What am I if my body does not work as it's supposed to?
Why did I have to be born this way?
I feel so lost, alone, and tired. I am beyond exhausted.
My life sucks with these horrible, painful periods every single damn month.
I can't stand it anymore. Everyone tells me it's normal.
It's not, I just know it!
How can I continue going on like this, with so much suffering all the time?
All I want is a baby!
Please, please, let me have a baby!
It's too much. I'm done with it all. If I can't have a baby, I just can't.

I need to accept the cards I have been dealt; it would be easier for everyone.
Maybe I'll "reshuffle the deck" somehow to be more in favor of what I want.
I need to just decide and commit to accepting myself for who I really am.
I need to move on with life.
Maybe I don't have to accept myself for who I am and make new, different choices and changes that could help.
GOD! I'm so sick of everything!

It pains me to know that these are sentiments that you are dealing with and facing every day of your life. I don't know exactly where you are in your journey, but wherever it is, I know all too well that it is a place where you repeatedly sink to the depths of your soul in painful ways, only to be wrapped in glazes of darkness, yet sustained by intermittent glimmers of renewed hope. This dichotomy can feel like an endless cycle for many of us.

As my journey continued through many, many years, my constant companions of frustration, pain, and suffering drowned me so many times. My brain continually asked, "Why on Earth am I experiencing this?" with the definition of "this" changing all the time.

I had to ask myself, do I accept the cards I have been dealt with? Or do I find ways to work the hell out of that hand? You, too, must ask this question. Do you accept the hand you were dealt and walk away? Or do you make the conscious, intentional choice to work the hell out of it?

Either way, **you are a warrior.**

A STARTING PLACE

A good place to start is to consider how much weight you are willing to carry around and are capable of handling. Most of us women innately know that we can carry a lot of weight but don't realize how resilient we truly are. We can learn to take ways and make choices that empower ourselves and help us to take control of our destiny. You have many choices. You can work with the cards you have got or not. You can also start one way and switch directions anytime if you like. And so, what if you make mistakes? You fall, rise, try again, make changes, accept, or run away. Either way, you will continue to be a warrior. Remember, dealing with endometriosis and gyno problems in different ways is hardcore shit. But you are a warrior. You can handle it. You need to remind yourself that no matter what you choose or don't choose to do, YOU ARE A WARRIOR!

On planet Earth, half of the population is female. The male has a slight lead, but it is pretty equal. Both females and males are important. We need both to reproduce our population, but the female has a bigger part to play. She can have a period every month, and she has the gift to carry a child for forty weeks. That equates to a lot more hormones, changes in her body, changes in her mood, and much more weight on the female's part compared to males.

Half of the population on Earth have periods, and more than 80 percent suffer from some form of discomfort during their period, according to many sources, including womens-health-concerns.org and the National Institute of Health. There are way too many women who suffer from PMS, heavy bleeding, cramps, cysts, migraines, breast tenderness, swollen bodies, and other period-related symptoms. Did you get that percentage? More than 80 percent of all women. That is insane!

That is way too many humans suffering **every month** for

over half of their lifetimes. I can't get why there is not more research, solutions, and support. We live in the twentieth century. Still, many girls and women hear from their mothers, friends, and doctors that the period is supposed to include pain, heavy bleeding, mood swings, and other discomfort. That is just how it is, and there is nothing to do about it. (Sigh!)

If the male population had to deal with these dynamics, there would be much more research by now, and many more working solutions and support provided for a long time already. We need to speak up more. With the advent of all the social media platforms, word is getting out much more than it used to, thank goodness. As we become even more empowered and assertive with our rights, we can continue to make positive changes that benefit all women globally. The bottom line is that horrible pain, discomfort, and suffering during a period is not normal. Our male population needs to step up a lot more to take responsibility, support, and take action in this matter. They don't live on their own planet! These problems affect them as well. Would they not like to see their loved ones, mothers, sisters, girlfriends, and wives feel better?!

Suffering during your period is not your fault. You haven't done anything wrong. You are a warrior every single month that you are dealing with this. But we forget that you have the right to feel alright every day, to feel beautiful, to be able to go to school or work every day, to enjoy activities every day, and to have an enjoyable social life. You don't have to feel awful or awkward every month. You don't have to, and you should not feel awful when you have your period.

We must stop what we have been programmed with for decades. It is time to change how females, males, and the world look at and treat periods. It is time that a woman gets support and pampering during her periods. It is time (since long ago) that women don't feel ashamed when they have their periods and that this is a subject we all can speak openly about. A period is normal, not shameful. Half of the population has a period every month, and still, there is so much hush, hush, hiding, speaking with a low voice, and not letting anyone know. Keep it a secret and, at the same time, just act as normal when your body is in pain, when you have cramps when you need to go to the restroom more often, and when you are afraid of leaking or smelling. Gosh, if anybody would notice, that would be awful, right? Wrong. A warrior does not accept such nonsense.

You don't have to live like this. There is support out there for you, and there are solutions that can ease your periods, your PMS, and the cramps you're suffering with every month of life. What we all can agree upon, though, is that it's time to redefine what a "normal" period really is. What we refer to as normal today is not what most women have to deal with twelve times a year, not to mention that you always get your period when there is something important or fun you need/like to do.

Take a minute to think about living in a society, having a school system, work, parents, partners, and friends who all have open minds when it comes to menstruation. Think about the idea of us living in a world where a period is something accepted as normal and beautiful. In this world, you are also allowed to take care of your body and attend to its unique needs when you have your period with the time off to get through it. What if your period was celebrated because your body is healthy and works as it is supposed to with the gift of creating life?

I think if the hush-hush and the pressure around periods goes down, the suffering goes down. What do you think? In today's life, we are supposed to be the same, with or without period. The period affects the body in many ways. In my dream world, I would like us to go back to nature. To follow the flow in our bodies. We need to listen to our bodies and what they need. I dream of a world where our periods are a part of life and not suffering for so many. With this book, I hope to open up to new ways to face your reality and find new solutions. I believe we must heal our bodies, minds, hearts, and souls first.

Medications or surgeries do not need to be the only and easy solution. If you have pain, it is easy to take a painkiller. We just want the pain to disappear so we can go on just like before. Painkillers are great sometimes. We need to be able to reduce pain. But today, that is a quick fix. We get pain, take a pill, and in less than thirty minutes, we feel great again. But the body is trying to tell you something. Your body wants you to listen. We can solve the pain for quite a long time with painkillers, but often, we must increase the intake of painkillers with time. We still do not listen to our own bodies, even if they speak louder. We are getting rid of the pain but not the cause. My intention with this book is to show many different approaches and ways to solve the cause of your pain and suffering. You deserve to feel the best you!

EVERY DAY, WEEK, MONTH, YEAR

This is your life. Are you ready to dive in and really listen to your body, mind, heart, and soul? Are you ready to find a sustainable lifestyle that will give you a more relaxed, less painful, and enjoyable life? It is possible. But nothing comes for free. It takes awareness, education, knowledge, and work. When you get the edge and know that you are over having this pain and suffering, you can make the conscious choice to find out what works for you, with the dedication required to also try many new things.

This book is a "smorgasbord" of ideas and solutions. Of course, there is much more out there that you can seek out to add to your knowledge repertoire. This book gives you a lot of options and ideas as a start. Maybe it will be enough for you, or maybe you dive into something else in parallel. The important thing is to find what works best for your body and your needs. The goal is to live a life without suffering and pain and possibly to find a way to have your baby. There is a lot of work to be done to achieve this. Remember, start the process, and then take it one step at a time.

MY BODY DOESN'T WORK RIGHT

Endometriosis, heavy bleedings, cysts, PCOS, or other gynecological challenges can make it more difficult to get pregnant and start a new life. More and more people start this journey with ART (Assisted Reproductive Technologies) or IVF (in vitro fertilization) and means supported fertilization. It is a way to assist in getting a pregnancy. Many women do not jump straight to an IVF treatment. Instead, they start with different treatments, hormones, and additional methods to support the fetus when a pregnancy appears.

Some good news is that in today's world, women do not have to suffer nearly as much from endometriosis, cysts, and other period-related pain compared to years ago. But, on the other hand, in today's world, the lifestyle we live with fast food, stress, and everything we do does affect us physiologically, with more and more people having difficulty getting pregnant on the first try. Many try for a long time.

Our desire to create a new life is an innate desire. It is in our DNA and genes to reproduce us. It does not matter if we are with our partner, on our own, or in a relationship with the same gender. Most women share the desire to have a little baby of their own to love, pamper, and cherish. It is insane how far we are willing to go to create and get that little life we long for.

I wish everyone who longs for a baby of their own can receive it. But I also would like you to fully understand what you will put your body, relationship, and whole life through while seeking this outcome. IVF or similar treatments are wonderful. It has helped many to get what they long for, but the golden coin has a backside. In this book, you will receive valuable information about the ups and downs during endometriosis and the IVF journey to create a new life. You will get to learn about what I went through to successfully have my twins. You will be able to experience firsthand what many other women have gone through to receive freedom from pain as well as to get pregnant. There will be many gems of things that you will consider for yourself if it suits you and your body. The truth behind many treatments and methods, like hormone treatments, will be shared with you. They definitely are not for everybody.

All the magical information bound together in this book will help you during critical decision-making times. Being under treatment to get pregnant is hard. Enduring horribly painful gynecological challenges suck.

No matter what you decide to do, no matter if you change directions hundreds of times or jump off the journey for a break or for good, either way, YOU ARE A WARRIOR! Do not ever forget that. I was a worrier for way too long, over decades, and I am worn out. I encourage you to see and embrace the warrior within yourself for this time of your life, help her step forward with respect, and tell her that this will not be forever.

As the warrior you are, embrace her, love her, and respect her. The warrior within you continues to figure things out, even when she is afraid, emotional, or irrational when she doubts, and even when she does not see a way out.

Remember:

She is extraordinary.

She is creative.

She is intelligent.

She is phenomenal.

She is confident.

She is kind.

Shared Heartbeats

She is important.
She is magical.
She is authentic.
She is amazing.
I am she. She is Me.
You are she. She is You.
Wishing you all the best in all you decide to do in life,
with my love and light,
from a Queen Warrior.

Chapter 2
Annika's Story

"Don't let anyone tell you that you can't do something. Especially not yourself."

— Mindy Kaling

W hen I was little, about five or six years old growing up in Sweden, I thought I would not have children of my own. My first memory of this idea came when my grandpa's sister retired and started working as a nurse in Africa taking care of little kids. That is when I thought I shouldn't have children on my own. Instead, I too would adventure off to Africa just like she did, to work and take care of the lovely children of Africa! This made me feel so joyful, full of love and excitement because by giving to all those little kids, I too will learn so much about another culture, country, language, and foods!

As time went by, I eagerly listened to all the stories from my grandaunt and always landed in the same place with my thinking: the idea that there just were too many children in the world already that were not being taken care of and not getting love or support. Will the world in my adult future even be a place where I would want children? I remember thinking about this a lot through-out my childhood. It became so ironic too because later in life, when I wanted to try to have children on my own, I had nothing but problems, pain, and suffering. When I was just a little girl, maybe I knew deep inside me that having children naturally and organically was not going to happen for me so I secretly kept a place in my heart for all the children in Africa.

Around age twelve, pamphlets, brochures and letters started being delivered to the house I was growing up in, in Sweden. They arrived in the mail with information about periods and advertising for different products like tampons or pads, with different companies providing free samples. I created a place in my bathroom with a basket in a drawer to keep all of them together. My mom and I didn't talk that much about "female stuff." She did tell me that someday, when I was going to the bathroom, I would find some red on my toilet paper or in the toilet and that I might feel some pain or discomfort in my belly. She told me that that is normal and that I should not think that I was sick. No one had told my mother about periods and so the pattern with me continued. My mom shared that she went to the bathroom one day, pulled down her underwear and there was blood spotted on them all over. Some red even dripped into the toilet. She cried and was scared thinking she was dying. Nobody had ever told my poor mother about periods: no sisters, aunties, moms, friends, teacher, or neighbors. What horrible fear and silence she lived in. How can something so normal make you feel so ashamed, wrong, and bad?

Talking about periods, having conversations early on and throughout childhood needed to be occurring and normalized for her so that this could have been done slowly with me! Reliable information should have been provided so that misconceptions, fears, triggers, and confusion are not experienced by a girl. This is how horrible stigmas, taboos and myths are started, perpetuated, and then experienced. I remember my mother always acting like everything was normal, even when she felt like crap. That was role modeled to me all my growing up years: fake it and wear a mask.

Hundreds of hormones were running through my adolescent body and I had constant cravings for chocolate and ice cream but couldn't talk about it. I started to lose my temper a lot as well. In Sweden, the grade five girls and boys go separately to learn about their body changes from the school nurses. When I approached becoming even more of an adolescent girl around the age of 13, my periods started coming and they were easy, but quickly, they leveled up and I started experiencing horrible symptoms that lasted for about a week. These symptoms, I would soon come to realize, were constant with every cycle I had. Unbeknownst to me, they would made their ugly return with every single cycle for the rest of my life. Pain was consistent, sometimes predictable, and sometimes varied with my ovulation and menstruation. As odd as it may sound, any of these negative patterns that developed gave me some comfort because I would at least be able to anticipate the next thing, giving me some twisted sense of control.

Having diminished sleep quality contributed to an increase in daily life problems. Symptoms of anxiety, depression, and especially negative self-talk/esteem were making their presence known and contributing to the start of mental health issues for me. Overall, I was living and surviving, but had a reduced quality of life. There clearly was disease present and damage starting to occur, but during my adolescence, none of this was known because no one talked about it.

I could handle school when I was on my period, but it was not easy. The pain and fear of leakage was just too much. I would rest in the bus on the way to school after challenging mornings of trying to get out of bed and get ready. I often arrived at school stressed and sweaty, I was sluggish and kind of out of it.

In my last year of high school, on a field trip that lasted several days, I got my period and had a hard time sitting on the bus seat. On our way home I asked to lay down and rest for a bit at the end row in the bus. My teacher told me that that was not appropriate. When we got back to school, I was called to the principal's office. It was so embarrassing to be called in from class to see the principal! The principal came to think that I was on drugs or hung over from alcohol. He would say things that suggested this to me. He said that these must be the reason (drugs and alcohol) for causing me to feel sick. This was completely beyond my comprehension because I got so good at keeping a poker face while I was in pain. It also helped that I repeatedly told myself that "the show must go on."

In addition to this horror, the principal was a male, handsome and known for being a cool guy. With all that aside, there was no way I could not tell him about my periods because I felt ashamed and embarrassed. During a typical school day, when I was on my period, I continued to need a lot of breaks due to the pain. The bathroom became a place of refuge for me where I felt safe. My eyes would close as I rested on top of the toilet seat, did some deep breathing, and gather up some energy. Looking back, I realize this was the beginning of my meditation practice. I was reluctant to speak up about my symptoms as I did not have the education, awareness or most importantly the confidence to talk about such things to my male principal or the teachers. Afterall, I was told by family, friends, and school nurses that *"periods are supposed to be painful with cramping."* How was I supposed to know the difference between "normal period pain" and "abnormal pain?" All my school peers seem to have been handling their periods just fine. I came to accept that the acute, chronic, insufferable pain that started taking over my life at age 13 was here to stay. What else was I supposed to do?

When I started my periods, I remember obsessing over the thought about why couldn't I have been a boy so none of this would be happening to me and I would be able to do whatever I wanted with no periods? I was so angry, and as time passed by, my anger increased. To help myself out, I promised myself I would never let my periods stop me from doing anything I wanted. Not Ever. I would always push through, no matter what. I would not let other people know that I "couldn't handle" them. I would rise above it all just as the high pile of stacked small pads rose higher and higher to protect my underwear. Even larger, thicker pads were added on top of the small pad pile to help absorb the heavy bleeding. Tampons were used in conjunction with the pads, having to change them every other hour. I would hide and sneak around with pads in every pocket available and stuffed my backpack full. I had to always be prepared. Needless to say, getting through high school was beyond challenging because most of the time I was debilitated.

PUBERTY AND THE PILL

Being much later in life now, I find myself asking, how did I really survive this teenage season of my life? I survived from several coping techniques that naturally developed. First of all, I would consciously acknowledge my debilitating pain, telling myself that there will be worse days than others and this wasn't going to last forever. Second, there was a lot of pervasive self-talk occurring in that brain of mine. Much of my mind's real estate was occupied with what I needed to do hour by hour of my life to get by. I would still try to keep up my social life, sometimes going to multiple parties in the same evening. I did not want to disappoint my friend group nor anyone in the church community. Last, I tried to get enough sleep and tried not feel guilty about taking naps any time I could. When I really needed it, I wish I could have what I call a "pajama day" to give myself a full day to rest, but this remained a pipe dream that never came true. This is so sad. I was Doris in Nemo, where I kept swimming along. "Just keep swimming. Just keep swimming...!"

Like many other young girls seeking relief from their premenstrual days and their periods, I went on the pill my last year of high school to help with the pain and heavy bleedings. I gained weight, had mood swings, bouts of irritability and frustration. But the pain got a bit less after starting a pill regime and my bleedings were reduced in heaviness. I set an alarm every morning to remember to take the pill because I quickly learned that if I didn't take the pill at the exact time every day, I would experience break through bleeding. If I took the pill even a couple of hours late, my body was so sensitive that it resulted in me having break through periods.

Originally, I had to try several different types of pills to find the best one for my body. It was when I was in high school studying tourism and travel as a subject that I had heard from the other girls about their birth control pill experiences.

I finally made an appointment in that city after I got called once again to the principal's office and was once again completely humiliated. It was a midwife nurse that took care of me for my first ob-gyn appointment that was not urgent. I went through a normal female medical appointment process and the midwife answered all my questions and explained a lot about birth control pills. I was eighteen at that time. I went to the pharmacy and collected the pills at once and started. In Sweden, birth control pills were something you must pay out of your own pocket. It was not expensive. I told my mom that I was starting birth control pills to see if it could help with my periods. This is when I first started feeling that my body was failing me. I felt ashamed and disappointed with my body.

When I was eighteen, I had my first serious boyfriend. I started to stay over at his place. One night, I was starting my period when I was there, my cramping prevented me from being able to sleep. I would move so much in his bed that I kept him up too, which forced him to sleep on the couch. He also tried to help me out by giving me "pain killers" to ease the pain. I was never really sure what it was he gave me as it seemed to affect my head and did nothing to numb my cramps. To this day, I wonder if it was really a pain killer. Romantic thoughts of intimate times together were ruined and becoming sporadic.

At the time, I was working at the front desk of an urgent care clinic. I had to go to work, no matter what. There were no other options. I was at his place that morning when my night kept him sleeping on the couch. I had so much pain that morning that I could hardly even walk. I was bent over in ninety degrees to be able to walk. Thank God I had to sit in a chair for my job. A nurse at the clinic noticed my discomfort, asked me some questions, and immediately sent me in to see the clinic doctor.

After a short discussion with this doctor, he sent me to see the ob-gyn at the local hospital. The ob-gyn was also male and I remember feeling triggered from my high school days, embarrassed especially when spreading my legs and insecure about the processes. It was here where I had my first ultrasound. I learned that this transvaginal ultrasound can show whether there is fluid behind the uterus and that fluids causes pain. A wand was placed into my vagina to take detailed ultrasound images. The ob-gyn explained to me that there was fluid behind my uterus, a lot of fluid with the most of it being blood. That was the information I got. He told me not to do exercises or anything heavy or physical during the three coming weeks and that my body would solve this situation by itself. I was freaked out! But kept myself together, as usual.

Many years later I learned that every time I bled, for my specific anomaly, it was common for the blood to flow up into my fallopian tubes and leak out to different parts of my body and was also getting stuck outside my uterus into my bowels and colon. As if that wasn't enough, this blood and other fluids were traveling to other parts of my body. I also learned that it was also common for small clots to form in different spots in my body. Tissue that would normally form inside my uterus would grow outside of my uterine cavity instead. The clots got stuck in different places and stayed there until my hormones changed during ovulation. Contractions came and went that were related to the blood clots" inflammation of the female areas. Eventually, my body was supposed to absorb all the fluids and blood, but old blood clots could linger on and bleed at later cycle times or be released when on my next period. They were disgusting. Bright red clumps or dark maroon-brown clumps would come out of my vagina as blobs onto my stack of napkins during a menstrual flow. The clots varied in size, texture, and consistency. The jelly like ones were the grossest.

This was all such a mess, I remember thinking. I was a mess. My periods were a mess and my life started to feel like a total mess. Why didn't I feel relieved knowing that the doctor had examined me and told me that I would be ok? Instead, I was over-whelmed and more depressed because I knew, deep within my soul, that I was not. What good did this do? I finally knew what was going on with my body and what was causing me so much suffering. In retrospect, it really was just another beginning, one where I was intimately familiar with all the gory details. I was experiencing what millions upon millions of women, generation after generation, experience. On top of it all, nobody takes your symptoms seriously and it takes a long time before you may even hear the word "endometriosis."

ROMANCE IN THE AIR

I eventually stopped the birth control pills, which coincided with me moving from Sweden to Germany. I worked in a restaurant in the evenings as well as a lot of overtime. The pain with my period remained the same but another difference started happening. I still remember the day when my menstrual blood had a big piece of tissue, almost looking like a nasty tumor growth encased with thin mucus membrane. I was scared. Nothing looked "normal" to me. The texture was made up of gross weird stuff I had never had before, which I later learned were parts of cysts that were dislodged in my uterus. I did not tell the family that I was working and living with when this change occurred or what I was experiencing. Cysts are a common by- product from endometriosis, I learned much later in life. But at this time, I still had not been diagnosed with endometriosis and certainly didn't know I had it. I was scared and actually thought I had a serious illness. By this time, the poker face was unable to make an appearance due to all the fear and pain. I spent four days in bed at the doctor's recommendation. My family thought it was some stomach issue and gave me toasted bread with butter and tea. Not much food! I let them think they were right.

I went back on a different pill to help with breakthroughs. The cyst tissues got a bit less after that. My next job was a ski instructor. This is when I started to notice that the more stress I put on my body, the sicker I got. The correlation was strong. That year alone, I got strep, other throat infections, colds, high fevers, flu, stomach illnesses and other viruses. These illnesses were on top of my horrible periods and they were connected. When my period started, an illness would hit me as well. I called it the "bonus package." My immune system was going downhill with every slope I skied, and my mother, for the first time in my life, started to show some concern.

I was at the age of twenty-five when I met my husband, Magnus, in Sweden at that ski area. I was in another relationship at the time I met him, but it was not a healthy one. I hadn't found the courage to break it off yet. It took me a couple of months to make this happen. I first saw Magnus in December and I broke up with my ex-boyfriend in February. I was holding a workshop for the Swedish Professional Ski School (SPS) for about fifty people. I was nervous, but it went wonderfully well. I didn't notice him then, yet he can tell me exactly what I was wearing the first time he set eyes on me!

The ski instructors had decided to have a bonfire one evening, and it was here that I heard him sing. WOW! He was good! I liked him from the first sight and sound of him singing at that beautiful bon fire. I began to see him out on the slopes. Occasionally we would accidentally meet at bars, discos and we always would dance with each other. We also started to play beach volley ball together and enter tournaments. I was the really good beach volleyball player and he was just a beginner. We used to joke that he had "Toblerone" candy arms! A romance was brewing and I soon knew that love was in the air because he would show up at my tournaments as a surprise, just to hang out with me. It was a new beginning for me where we were discovering what we had in common and what we enjoyed together. This became an important component of our falling in love. One special evening we went down to the beach, had a long talk, and ended the evening with our first kiss. I had fallen for him.

That fall, I had to honor a contract that I had already signed for an au pair job in Switzerland. Sadly, we all had to leave that little ski resort and town and return to our other lives. During the six months I was in Switzerland, he (my new boyfriend!) came and visited me twice. We had so much fun together and I realized that he was caring, fun, gentle and made me laugh. I was feeling the best I had in many years, emotionally and regarding self-esteem. He adored me and my body.

When I came back from Switzerland, I moved in with him in his study apartment. It was a bit scary. It went a bit fast but when you know you know! After two years we found a bigger apartment and it felt great to have our first home that we had chosen together. We had a social life, as well as many activities we enjoyed together. He was always wonderful to me, and did things for me, saying small things that makes a girl happy and affectionate. We dated for about a year and then lived together for six years. I worked a lot during those years, participated to the best of my ability in different sports, attended parties, and engaged in a lot of traveling.

For the next two years, everything continued happening to me gynecologically as it had been the previous eight years. I had tried many different birth control pills to help with my chronic female problems. I did hear of a shot that could be taken every three months, in lieu of a pill for birth control and decided to give that a try. I was desperate to find relief from the bleedings and pain again. I learned that a colleague of mine was getting injections that reduced her menstrual bleedings, so, I looked into it. I started getting these injections from the midwife and my periods went away, 100%. Unfortunately, soon afterward, I learned from one of my aunts, who also was a midwife in another Swedish region, that these shots were not being given to women before they had children because there were too many health risks. In fact, it was banned in the region of Sweden she worked in. I had such contradicting feelings when I learned of this. After the first shot, my period didn't come back for two whole years. This was shocking, but also provided a great relief for me to have some healing. During this time, my relationship with my boyfriend Magnus blossomed and we became serious. We decided to get married! I was thirty years old.

MARRIED LIFE

What a beautiful honeymoon! I was able to go about life untethered, free, and unburdened. We had planned a four-week honeymoon around Christmas. We left before Swedish Lucia, December 13 and traveled all the way to Philippines where we hid away in a little dive resort. We ventured into Malaysia and Thailand as well. It was wonderful! Lovely weather, lots of diving and great food. We had sex every day, at least once, except for the five days when I got my first period after more than two years without it. We were hoping to get pregnant during our honey moon. We even talked about what our baby would look like. I had so many thoughts and dreams about what our baby would look like, being that s/he would have features of both of us. These visions would blow my mind and became obsessive. Everything felt so right and in place for me for the first time in my life. We were fully enjoying everything together and experiencing the natural order of the next phase of our life.

Unfortunately, this short time of happiness did not last long because when we returned from our honeymoon, after only two days off, I started a new job along with both of us starting to refurbish our apartment. The real kicker was that I started my period that exact same week: my horrid period, the new job, our apartment refurbishing efforts and just back from honeymoon. It was at this time that I fully realized the correlation between the roles of my life stressors with the start of a new bleeding. They exacerbated each other tremendously. When you are "in a situation," going through many life experiences simultaneously, we women tend to stay so busy pushing through all the stress that we don't realize how much stress we really are under at the time. This was my second period after the two years without one, and it lasted for three long, bloody weeks. What should have been the beginning of our new life together as one of the best years of my life ended up being one of the most miserable because every period after that lasted for weeks, with only few days off in between. This became my new way of living in horror for four long years.

The apartment we were renovating as our new place would have all that we wanted. There was a cute, cozy loft with balcony and a hot tub. We had been looking around for more than a year prior to our honeymoon to find this apartment. It actually was the attic of a five-level building with a loft. With help from our dads and friends, we put up walls and built the apartment out. During this whole time, I experienced long periods with short times in between. It was strenuous on my body, to say the least. But I was determined to not let others know that I was suffering in the least bit even though I was weak, tired, and stressed out. Hiding my emotions continued to be a habit I was good at. Looking back, I realize how isolating this was for me, how lonely it made me feel and just how wrong it was in so many ways.

There were many trips to the hardware store to choose what we liked for the floors, carpets, and walls. I wish I could have immersed myself more into this whole process, but as long as I wasn't leaking, all was well. I really did not disagree with what my husband wanted. In fact, we really didn't disagree on many things and made a great team! As the days and months passed, I was falling deeper and deeper in love with my husband. This is what sustained me. This is what lifted me up. This is what living is truly about: love. We continued on having so much fun building our own home.

It took us six months to renovate the loft/attic apartment in that big house, but we made the apartment our home. We built the walls, painted, did everything that was required to make a beautiful living space. I poured myself into this project as much as I could. It was a melding of loving efforts between Magnus and I, our friends and family as well. It was a love project. Even though my bleedings were horrible, I kept returning to that teenage promise I made to myself to keep moving through life and pushing through no matter how painful it was. It really was a testament to how much we humans can endure. Mind you, it wasn't like being a prisoner of war or anything of that magnitude, but in some ways, I was a prisoner.

These four years of my life were some of the most dreaded and longest years with glimmers of sparkling happiness dripped throughout. The closest people to me always told me that I was a positive person, even if they knew I was going through a hard time. But to me, unless a person authentically feels positive from their heart, versus telling themselves and making themselves be positive in a fake manner, it is not genuine positivity. I was still faking it. I was going through my life with a mask on because of the shame. I felt ashamed. I was not good enough.

By my thirty-first birthday, everything was just a mess. I continued having heavy, heavy bleedings. I stopped the shot before I got married in April. In the fall, I thought several times that maybe I was pregnant because my breasts were tender. I wasn't pregnant though. For many of the following months I felt breast tenderness, but no periods. When I finally got my periods back, they didn't stop. They just prolonged. Hemorrhaging went on for almost three hundred days during a year. Yes, 300! Sometimes it was just a few drops, sometimes it was heavy. This continued for the coming years until I turned thirty-four. I later learned that this condition is called "menorrhagia."

I was working for a school during this time. I looked pale a lot and knew it because this old school nurse was a bit worried for me and would stare at me, telling me outright that I was pale. One day she changed it up a bit. She actually said to me that I looked like a ghost! I was astonished because that exact morning, I had applied extra make up to make myself to try and look better. So much for that effort. I wasted money just to be invisible! What irony.

HORMONES & PAIN KILLERS

This period was different for me though, as I felt and knew I was losing too much blood. Just like so many other times before in my life, I decided to give another ob-gyn a try during this time. She had me try different pills to reduce the heavy bleedings, as well as putting me on new hormones to try to balance my cycle. I also got strong pain killers, which turned into even stronger pain killers as time went by. I was on a pretty slippery slope. Soon, these pain killers were just under the morphine levels. I started using heating pads and added drinking some alcohol as well. I slowly faded into a numbing stage.

I woke up one morning in so much pain, I admitted myself to the hospital. This is about the time when my husband started working longer hours several days of the week. He was avoiding coming home just find me at another doctor's office, in the hospital or in bed all the time with heating pads and a buzz. The buzz starting coming when I combined a pain killer with a glass of red wine. Cheers to me! He felt helpless and unable to help. Years afterward, he told me he could not take coming home and seeing me all curled up in a ball on the bed in a baby pose, crying, sad and in pain. Needless to say, we drifted apart, became like roommates, and only talked about practical things. There was nothing we could do to end this nightmare. Filled with much sadness, my husband rarely shared his ideas of new solutions any more. Instead, he focused on the domestic side of tasks like grocery shopping, cooking, and laundry. He wanted to invite friends over, but my body was too exhausted. He zoned out because he couldn't take seeing me so sad and in pain. All the while, I was consumed with the thought of him leaving me. Shame and fear were not a winning combination, especially for a woman who was barely surviving survival mode.

Chapter 3
Ways to Enjoy this Book

"Speak your mind – even if your voice shakes."

— Maggie Kuhn

First of all, I want to thank you for choosing to read this book. I know you are struggling, feeling sad, a bit mad and maybe depressed and out of solutions. I know and hope this book will give you hope, tools, and solutions that make your journey easier and smoother. Having a hard time with periods, endometriosis, not getting pregnant, and experiencing hormone or IVF treatment is a lot to take in. It is a lot for your body, mind, and heart to carry. I get it. I've been there and gotten to the other side. My book is here to be your trusting guide while you are on your journey.

While reading this book, you will find information about my journey, many different treatments, a lot about medicine from both the academic world and holistic, and many holistic and alternative methods that I tried. I still use and enjoy several of the holistic and alternative treatments. When your life does not follow your plans, things get in your way, and you get frustrated and lose the patience to deal with everything. My hope is that this book can support you in finding your path to a healthy life with joy and balance.

Please take a moment to ask yourself what your goal is and what you are willing to do to get there. This is what I mean by that. Are you willing to invest time, money, partnership, communication, treatments, hormones, IVF, and other things that can occur during this journey? Especially your time? What do you think will be your reality in six months, one year, two years? It is a great way to start becoming more familiar with what you feel and where your limits are. Ask your partner to do the same, and then you can share what you think and feel with each other. Of course, you can change your mind during the journey, but to know where you both are right now is a great start and critical to fully embracing where it is you want to go.

So, here are some of the lessons I have learned. I don't recommend jumping too quickly into different treatments in hopes of getting what you want quickly. Set a practice to always do research before you start on a new path or beginning a new process. This whole experience is about your body, your life, the life you want to bring into this world, and, most importantly, honoring what you feel is right for you. Maybe you need more time than you think to reach your goal. Maybe less time will be needed, but no matter what, time is going to pass. Prepare yourself. Pamper yourself. Prepare your partner. Pamper your partner. Prepare your relationship. Pamper your relationship, and do this over and over again through your journey.

If you feel lost and don't know where to start, my intention is that this book will help you by being a guide and a place where you can reflect, think things through, and even contact me directly for support. When I experienced my journey, I didn't know who to talk to, where to find the best recommendations, how to navigate through all that was happening to me. My body was failing me, or so I thought in my mind for so many years. I lost self-confidence. At one point, my relationship with my husband deteriorated and plummeted to much less communication and much less taking care of each other. All those different things that pop up while you are going through life and you don't know what to do or where to turn to with your concerns, my book will be here for you.

My wish is that you find a lot of resources to make your journey smoother, easier, and more joyful. In this book, you will find resources and tools to go step by step through your process. I have shared so many experiences and included the hard stuff for you and your loved ones to learn from in an easy, friendly way. I will show you how I recovered from my journey so you can, too. You are here because you feel lost and need support with many challenges to living the life you desire. You deserve to feel and truly know in your heart that you are not alone. Your body is wonderful, and you can help it heal and to provide for you what you need from it. This book will help you with the suffering you have been experiencing and guide you to a healthy, balanced life of joy. There will be exercise and activities to assist you in your healing.

Here are some of the ways in which you can experience this book:

OPTION 1: Read this book for yourself, front to back, in chronological order.

Choose this option specifically for yourself if you:

- Are searching for an easy way to get a lot of information on endometriosis, IVF, and different alternative treatments.

- Feel that you are alone, find yourself having trouble with your periods, or struggle with fertility.
- Anow you want to better understand the different steps of the ways but don't know where to start.
- Are not drawn to a specific chapter, start on page one.
- Feel a need to be motivated and start moving toward your goal and healing.
- Have a need to find some more information to be better prepared at a doctor's visit or to talk to your partner.
- Are the partner or the support person who wants to understand what your loved one is going through to increase your empathy and compassion skills
- Want to support yourself, your friend, or your daughter experiencing heavy periods, unbearable cramping, and a deep fear of those days each month.

OPTION 2: Choose your order.

Choose this option to experience this book if you:

- Are drawn to a certain chapter or topic and feel a need to start with that information.
- Would like to know more about another person's journey to help yourself.
- Are a support person for someone who is dealing with heavy bleedings, cramps, days at home from school or work, hormone treatments, or IVF, and you just want specific ways to support your loved ones.
- Feel the need to find an activity, tool, or exercise to support your situation, the feelings and thoughts that are over you.

OPTION 3: Chunk it out.

Choose this option if you:

- Are overwhelmed and only can take in small parts at one time.
- Have little time, here and there, and can only read for a short period at time.
- If you have some time when you are in the bathroom or in the tub!

OPTION 4: Read it with your partner or friend.

This approach is a special, intimate way to journey through this book with another person. Consider this option if you:

- Want to embrace this journey together as a couple or with a supporting friend.
- Like to talk through what you read.
- Like the idea of taking turns reading out loud to each other.
- Communicate with post-it notes. (You can put them on the pages that you like and share what you think about it and why.)
- Like journaling together. You can keep and share the same journal, or each have your own journals.

I wish I could tell you that this process will be smooth and easy with no hard, brutal work. I wish I could also tell you that everything will happen so quickly, like a fairy waving a magic wand and putting a quick fairy spell over you, but we both know that's not going to happen. The truth is that you need to invest all your resources—time, money, and energy—and be willing to change in many ways. But, with this understanding early on in your processes and applying many of the tips and tricks shared in this book, you will be closer to what you are longing for!

With help from this book, you will safely navigate your healing journey to hopefully reach your desired goal. You will experience your inner critic, your ego that wants to judge you, talk bad to you, and be mean to you. Try to ignore that voice. Focus on listening to your heart and trusting in yourself and your own body. Focus on being honest with what you have experienced and will experience, and have an open mind to the process. This, too, shall pass. One day, you will find yourself on the other side, and that day, you will look back and be proud of yourself for listening to your heart and knowing you did your best in every decision, treatment, exercise, or whatever you choose to follow. I have experienced a long process and have hit many big bumps in the road. But somehow, I believed that from all the bleeding, pain, treatments, surgeries, needles, blood draws, fear, studying, and education, I have learned a lot and grown exponentially.

My deepest wish is for you to find a lot of information, tools, exercises, support, help, relief, and joy reading this book and start to prepare for your journey in a most confident manner. You are beautiful in every way. You are a miracle on a journey of a miracle. Take care of your mind, body, heart, and soul. They all make up your blessed temple, and are your best friends. Give them love, patience, care with grace.

Chapter 4
Knowledge is Power

"Doubt is a killer. You just have to know who you are and what you stand for."

— Jennifer Lopez

Knowledge is power. It gives you strength and courage. Knowledge is also a form of empowerment by making you more confident in your choices and decisions. The more you learn and know regarding any topic, the more confidence and self-advocacy you will have. In this chapter, I will share knowledge on many gynecological diseases and other critical topics to get you started on your journey of self-knowledge about your body and the possible challenges. Move forward on your own to do deeper research on any topic you need to.

To gain knowledge, you need to invest in yourself through research and make this a priority! You can find a lot of information in books and online, as well as by talking with people. I encourage you to do all the research you can to feel confident about your unique situation and challenges along the way, as well as any specific topic you feel unsure about. Becoming knowledge-able will also put you on a level that allows you to have more meaningful conversations with your medical team and make informed decisions.

There will be so many decisions to make throughout your journey. Decisions about how you will take care of and treat your body, what procedures you should have, what medications you agree you should be taking, and the schedules associated with hormone treatments. Decisions about how much money to spend on everything, as well as decisions about when enough is enough. The more knowledge you have prior to making a decision, the better decisions you will make for yourself.

I regret not becoming more knowledgeable much earlier in my life. My research and knowledge-seeking should have started when my horrible periods began. It unfortunately remains so sad and upsetting that so many girls and women continue suffering in today's contemporary times from severe problems related to their periods. If this was a cyclical problem being suffered by men, much more research would have been done historically, and more support would have been given. Also, if this was happening to men, many of the typical female reproductive problems would already be solved. But men don't have the issues we have, so most of this is not prioritized in the medical research community.

We need much more support, help, and ways to alleviate women's suffering and pain. How is this accomplished? Through knowledge. Knowledge is power. Become your own health advocate, and don't settle for anything less than what satisfies you.

The other aspect of women's suffering that remains upsetting is how many women see many doctors but don't receive a diagnosis or relevant help. It usually takes five to eight years to get a diagnosis in cases where painful periods exist. For me, it took twenty-five years—**twenty-five years!** There are way too many other women around the globe who have a similar story to mine. It is a shame. I wish for a much brighter future with more understanding, support, and knowledge.

Today, the most typical recommendation you get from an ob-gyn when you go in for an appointment for horrible period pains is to go on birth control pills as a first step. Then, it is also common that you get the suggestion of some type of surgery as another option to get rid of the period problem. So, the pill to start you off and then surgery as options. There are so many more ways to help yourself. How do I know? Through knowl-edge. With the latest research, we have a lot of advanced infor-mation on how to work with our bodies and not against them by using our food as medicine, through movement, employing alter-native treatments, and inner work to heal us in the most tremen-dous ways! Stay open-minded, gain knowledge, and forge forward.

PMS: PREMENSTRUAL SYNDROME

Established studies show that an estimated 90% of females of reproductive age are impacted in their lives by mild to acute premenstrual symptoms and pains. In Sweden, my home coun-try, more than 75% of all women suffer from PMS. Women expe-rience physical, psychological, and emotional suffering each month of their lives, starting around the age of twelve and well into midlife. PMS includes more than two hundred different symptoms that normally begin sometime after ovulation and dissipate shortly after the period starts. Symptoms may include a bloated belly, fatigue, sleep difficulties, tender breasts, irritation, frustration, anxiety, anger, and feeling low. Many people joke about PMS or may suggest that PMS exists only in a woman's head, but the experience is real and can be debilitating. PMS involves many aspects of female physiology, like hormones and neurotransmitters. I dream of a time when there is no such thing as PMS. Women have suffered too long, and we deserve a life without repeated, monthly suffering.

PMS starts with more minor symptoms that increase the closer a female is getting to her period. Some doctors will give you birth control pills or anti-depressive pills that may help. This may be the path you choose, but only do so if you are confident that you have all the knowledge you need to make this choice. Knowledge is power. If this is not the chosen path, maybe you will choose to balance the unbalanced hormones in your system. Or maybe you find out that you suffer specifically from dysmenorrhea. Dysmenorrhea is mainly caused by an unbalance in prostaglandins, and PMS is more caused by an imbalance from inflammation. How will you know the difference and which one pertains to you? The answer is, through knowledge.

In what other ways can we gain productive knowledge to help us through this journey? By learning about our habits and our stressors. Start by learning to understand your emotional strains along with your diet. Why do I point out both of these at the same time? Because what you are eating greatly impacts your emotional state. If you are eating like crap, you will not feel as good emotionally.

Many people have their own awareness or definition of stress. It is imperative that you understand, through this entire journey, what your stress levels are, what triggers your stress, and most importantly, how you can manage it. For instance, there are outward stressors that you can identify easily. Did you know there is such a thing as inward, unconscious stressors as well? These are much more difficult to identify and work with. They consist of things such as using too much social media, being on the computer/blue screens for far too long, and the constant interruptions of our cellular devices, all affecting your parasympathetic nervous system. Also, look at your stress levels around work and home workload. You may be enduring a lot of unconscious stress that needs to be removed to feel better. Today's life is so fast, and we must do so much more than before. Based upon my experience, thirty years ago, identifying all my stressors, inward and outward, was a lot easier because we did not have these electronic platforms along with social media. You could not be reached or interrupted all the time, 24/7. There was a true blessing and luxury in this way of life. Stepping back to nature to rethink how you are living, what you are doing, and how it impacts your life is a recommended activity I propose to you. Taking time to do this will enable you to reduce some of your bodily symptoms, get better sleep, come to terms with the changes you know you need to make for a much healthier lifestyle, and always know that I am here for you if working with me to help you navigate through all of this is something you would like.

I have outlined above and below many of the gynecological diseases that I have experienced, their symptoms and how to go about getting them diagnosed. Please remember, too, that the word disease can be broken down into two parts. "Dis" is a prefix that means "not" or "opposite of." Ease means to be easy, to flow without strain, and not to be difficult. Therefore, you can easily understand that the following are truly "dis-eases," and it is my goal to heal and bring the "ease" back into your life. This is a small list of chronic diseases, ones that I have experience with. There is a lot more on each topic and on other gynecological diseases for you to learn by doing additional research. Remember, knowledge is power.

ENDOMETRIOSIS

There are many common symptoms of the chronic disease known as endometriosis. They can include the following:

- Heavy periods
- Painful periods (dysmenorrhea)
- Pelvic pain
- Irregular periods
- Constipation
- Diarrhea
- Discomfort when peeing or bowel movement during periods
- Bloating or Nausea
- Painful intercourse
- Infertility
- Depression or anxiety
- Fatigue or low energy

When you suffer from many of the above symptoms, it could be endometriosis. If you suspect this, your doctor can follow patterns and do an ultrasound to try to find out if you have endometriosis. The only way to find out is to do a laparoscopy to diagnose it accurately. Laparoscopy is when the doctor checks your reproductive organs from the inside via peephole surgery. This is important because you need to fully understand your body and what you are potentially dealing with to manage it correctly.

If you are indeed diagnosed with endometriosis, the doctor normally recommends birth control pills because that often bring down the bleeding. The more bleeding you have, the harder it is on the body. The period blood can leak backward into other areas of the body like the stomach area, around your reproductive organs, bowls and even up to diaphragm and lungs. This blood that is supposed to remain in your uterus to be expelled during your period can also build up to create clots. This clot condition can worsen, too, the longer you have them. Unfortunately, with every period, more clots can build up, which only makes your cramps and suffering worse. That is why the doctor wants to reduce your bleeding. If you have a lot of clots, it only makes getting pregnant that much more difficult in the long term. With a traditional treatment, the doctor normally recommends pills that are special to specifically reduce your bleeding. Also, birth control pills or other hormones can assist in reducing the bleeding. You have to choose what is the best path forward for you.

There are other ways to support and heal your body from this hormone imbalance because endometriosis is essentially an imbalance in your body. Under the alternative treatments outlined later in this chapter, you can find information about other paths to follow. It is your body, and you'll make the best decision for you, not the doctor, not your spouse, not your family.

To help you see patterns and to keep track of your cycle and periods, I recommend a journal. You can use a traditional year calendar on paper or on your phone. Write down the start and end days of your periods. Make some notes on how each day was. Dark blood or light red, heavy or not, cramps or headache, and other symptoms. That will help you see patterns and returning symptoms. It is a great help and support when you see your ob-gyn regularly. You will receive a lot of helpful information and support. It is great to go back and see how it was a couple of months ago and see some changes as you try different lifestyle approaches, like moving more or eating healthier.

The more data you keep track of, the more you will know. It does not have to be a long, detailed story each day if you don't have time for that approach. You can have some symbols so you know what you mean, and that makes your writing fast. One way is to print a sheet to just fill out with your specific symptoms. That's what I did. You can copy my example below. It is a suggestion. Use what is relevant for you and easy to do to keep track. You may even come up with better ideas for keeping track of and following your body. You can buy a book that is specific to charting. I would love to hear about your experience. We can work together, and I can help you, provide support, and celebrate your progress.

TRACKING SHEET SUGGESTIONS

- Include the start and end dates of your period.
- Add your blood description (red, dark, heavy, light clumps).
- Add information on your body symptoms (cramps, pain level, headaches, nausea, dizzy).
- Keep track of how fatigued you are.
- Notice what kind of emotions are you experiencing (anxiety, sad, anger).

EASY TRACKING SHEET EXAMPLE

DATE: _________

	Red	Dark	Heavy	Light	Clumps	
BLOOD						

	Cramps	Pain 0-10	Headache	Nausea	Dizzy	Emotional
BODY						

Maybe you suffer from several of these symptoms and want to find the best treatment. Since treatments will work differently for individual women with endometriosis You should be aware of the different kinds of treatments, and their possible affects and side effects or complications. A combination of treatments can be said to assist in relieving the symptoms. There are several myths around endometriosis, and I heard several of them and believed in some of them.

SOME ENDOMETRIOSIS MYTHS

- The pain you're experiencing is normal. Get used to it.
- Endometriosis (endo) only affects your uterus, no other female "parts."
- Pregnancy cures endo.
- A full or partial hysterectomy cures endo.
- Endo means infertility.
- Endo is cured by birth control pills.
- If you have a little or minimal endo, you will only have mild symptoms.

The effect of endo is inflammation, formation of scar tissues, and adhesion. This horrible disease can block the fallopian tubes when growths cover the ovaries and cause problems in your intestines and bladder. If you have one or several of the endo symptoms, you have probably already seen a doctor. If not, get to one. Maybe you have seen several doctors, and nobody could help you. Don't fret! That is quite common, unfortunately. You can hear different ideas about what you are suffering from from many different doctors, but it still normally takes about five to seven years on average to get your correct diagnosis.

I recommend you contact the endometriosis association in your country. Most countries have an endometriosis association. There, you can find support and help with what to expect at a doctor's visit, questions you must ask, and what you can demand for support. The endometriosis association's goal is to support women with endo, spread the knowledge, and act for better health care. About 11% of people born with a uterus have endometriosis. That is about 190 - 200 million women and girls on the globe! That is way too many.

The following are excerpts echoed throughout many accredited articles I pulled from a Google search from credible sources. Continue doing your own research as well:

- Endometriosis is a chronic disease associated with severe, life-impacting pain during periods, sexual intercourse, bowel movements and/or urination, chronic pelvic pain, abdominal bloating, nausea, fatigue, and sometimes depression, anxiety, and infertility.
- There is currently no known cure for endometriosis, and treatment is usually aimed at controlling symptoms.
- Access to early diagnosis and effective treatment of endometriosis is important but is limited in many settings, including in low- and middle-income countries.

Endometriosis grows with the help of estrogen. By reducing estrogen, the body has a chance to slow down the diseases. This is why you get the recommendation of birth control pills and other hormone treatments. If you do not like or feel bad when taking birth control pills, I suggest you try alternative methods first to help your body and hormone levels balance.

PCOS – POLYCYSTIC OVARY SYNDROME

Based on my research with multiple sources, this is the common knowledge around PCOS, much of it derived from Mayo Clinic as the source: Polycystic ovary syndrome (PCOS) is a problem with hormones that happens during the reproductive years. If you have PCOS, you may not have periods often. Or you may have periods that last many days. You may also have too much of a hormone called androgen in your body.

With PCOS, many small sacs of fluid develop along the outer edge of the ovary. These are called cysts. The small fluid-filled cysts contain immature eggs. These are called follicles. The follicles fail to regularly release eggs. The exact cause of PCOS is unknown. Early diagnosis and treatment, along with weight loss, may lower the risk of long-term complications such as type 2 diabetes and heart disease. Symptoms of PCOS often start around the time of the first menstrual period. Sometimes symptoms develop later after you have had periods for a while.

The symptoms of PCOS vary. A diagnosis of PCOS is made when you have at least two of these:

- **Irregular periods -** Having few menstrual periods or having periods that aren't regular are common signs of PCOS. So is having periods that last for many days or longer than is typical for a period. For example, you might have fewer than nine periods a year. And those periods may occur more than thirty-five days apart. You may have trouble getting pregnant.
- **Too much androgen -** High levels of the hormone androgen may result in excess facial and body hair, called hirsutism. Sometimes, severe acne and male-pattern baldness can also happen.
- **Polycystic ovaries -** Your ovaries might be bigger. Many follicles containing immature eggs may develop around the edge of the ovary, and the ovaries might not work the way they should.

PCOS signs and symptoms are typically more severe in people with obesity. Factors that might play a role are low-grade inflammation and insulin resistance. If you suffer from PCOS, these are some difficulties you might have:

- Infertility
- Gestational diabetes or pregnancy-induced high blood pressure
- Miscarriage or premature birth
- Nonalcoholic steatohepatitis — a severe liver inflammation caused by fat buildup in the liver
- Metabolic syndrome — a cluster of conditions including high blood pressure, high blood sugar, and unhealthy cholesterol or triglyceride levels that significantly increase your risk of heart and blood vessel (cardiovascular) disease
- Type 2 diabetes or prediabetes
- Sleep apnea
- Depression, anxiety, and eating disorders
- Cancer of the uterine lining (endometrial cancer)

Obesity commonly occurs with PCOS and can worsen complications of the disorder. There is no cure for PCOS, but treatments that can support feel better. It is individual from woman to woman what may help. Again, I suggest trying to balance your body with food, exercise, rest, change of thoughts, and enough sleep. I have never been diagnosed with PCOS, but of course, I can relate to some of the symptoms.

CYSTS

The Mayo Clinic and John Hopkins University medicine have a lot to share regarding this topic: Ovarian cysts are more common in the childbearing years between puberty and menopause and less common after menopause. Taking fertility drugs often causes the development of multiple follicles (cysts) in the ovaries. These cysts most often go away after a woman's period or after a pregnancy.

OVARIAN CYST SYMPTOMS

Most ovarian cysts are small and don't cause any problems. Cysts more often cause trouble when they get bigger. So, what does an ovarian cyst feel like? Most of the time, they don't feel like anything at all. If you do have symptoms, signs of an ovarian cyst might include:

- Pelvic pain or pressure
- Dull ache in your back
- Bloating or feeling full
- Nausea
- Swelling in your belly area
- Pain during sex
- Pain during your period
- A frequent urge to pee or poop.

The ovarian cyst pain location may be on one side of your lower belly or in your back. Ovarian cyst pain may be sharp or dull, and it can come and go. Most cysts go away on their own, but you may need to see a doctor if your cyst grows large, causes symptoms, or bursts.

BURST OVARIAN CYST SYMTOMS

A cyst can break open or rupture. You'll probably feel some pain when this happens, but you might not. You may notice some discomfort a few days after your cyst bursts, too. Sometimes, when ovarian cysts rupture, you'll have discharge that looks like vaginal spotting or bleeding.

Symptoms of a burst ovarian cyst may include:

- Sharp, sudden pain in your lower belly or back
- Bloating that doesn't go away
- Abnormal spotting or bleeding

Ovarian cysts are common. Most of the time, you have little or no discomfort, and the cysts are harmless. Most cysts go away without treatment within a few months. But sometimes ovarian cysts can become twisted or burst open (rupture).

FOUR COMMON TYPES OF CYSTS

1. Corpus luteum cysts. The corpus luteum is what's formed after your ovary releases an egg.
2. Follicular cysts. A follicle in your ovary is responsible for releasing an egg during ovulation.
3. Endometriomas. Endometriomas are cysts that form out of endometrial tissue.
4. Dermoid cysts are solid or fluid-filled sac or pocket within or on the surface of an ovary.

Endometriomas are cystic lesions that stem from the disease process of endometriosis. Endometriomas are most commonly found in the ovaries. They are filled with dark brown endometrial fluid and are sometimes referred to as "chocolate cysts." The presence of endometriomas indicates a more severe stage of endometriosis.

I have had many cysts. Many of them have been extremely painful. I guess they were mostly chocolate cysts that ruptured by themselves. I have had clear cysts as well. I can't recall how many times I went straight to the ob-gyn doctor with acute, severe pain. It normally takes some hours or a night before you can see the doctor. Often, when I arrived, the pain had released a bit, and the only thing the doctor could see on ultrasound was fluid in the stomach. That is painful, but the body "cleans it up" in a couple of days. My fourth surgery was when a big cyst, about 5.6 cm in diameter, was attached to the ovary, stomach wall, and bowels.

For several months, it oscillated between being small and then big, with the cycle of horrible pain coming and going. I went to urgent care when I got pain down to my knee, and my stomach was swollen. The doctor was not so concerned about the cyst. They were more concerned that my bowels were full. I had only been able to poop "wiener sausages" for a long time but did not pay attention to that. In less than three weeks, I had surgery to remove the cyst. They wanted to perform the surgery earlier, but I needed to take care of some private arrangements first. I was used to bad pain, some days more or less. This was my first surgery with a robot. A robot makes it easier for the doctor to work with smaller tools. I did not notice any difference in pain or stitches after compared to a normal surgery.

WHAT IS INFERTILITY?

Infertility, or not being able to get pregnant after trying for one year, can be difficult for individuals and couples to go through. Infertility is fairly common, and it can even mean getting pregnant but having stillbirths or miscarriages. Let's look at some infertility statistics to better understand what it is and how it affects people.

Infertility is the inability to get pregnant even after having frequent and unprotected sex for one year. Infertility can affect both men and women and is usually self-diagnosable by an inability to get pregnant. Some women may also have a menstrual cycle that's too long or too short, and having certain health problems like pelvic inflammatory disease or uterine fibroids may predispose someone toward being infertile. Doctors can run many kinds of tests to help determine what might be causing fertility problems for an individual or couple. Transvaginal ultrasounds can help detect possible uterine abnormalities, blood tests can look for abnormal hormone levels, and semen analysis can detect semen abnormalities in men that might be playing a role in infertility. Infertility treatments are always improving, and many people are eventually able to successfully conceive. How common is infertility? Based on my research, the World Health Organization (WHO) has the following to share.

According to WHO, about sixty to eighty million couples worldwide have infertility. Southern and Eastern Europe and East Asia have some of the lowest fertility rates, with 1.5 children per woman. On average, one in four couples in developing countries experience infertility. 2023 was a low point in Sweden for the number of children born. It has not been as low since 2003. The number of children born between January and March 2023 in Sweden was the lowest in twenty years. Fertility is the lowest in fifty years in many countries worldwide. Germany and the USA are about the same as in previous years. Here are some more fun facts:One in four healthy women in their 20s and 30s will get pregnant during any single menstrual cycle (American College of Obstetrics and Gynecologists, 2018).

- One in ten healthy women in their 40s will get
  pregnant during any single menstrual cycle
  (American College of Obstetrics and Gynecologists,
  2018).

- In general, fertility begins to decrease for most women more quickly after the age of 35. (American Society for Reproductive Medicine 2012).
- Couples in which the male partner is forty years or older are more likely to have difficulty conceiving. (CDC 2019).
- Sperm quality generally does not become a problem for men until after the age of 60. (American Society for Reproductive Medicine 2012).

COST OF INFERTILITY TREATMENTS

All treatment costs for infertility can range from $5,000 to $73,000 USD. A single treatment costs around $3,000 to $5,000. There are packages and different options depending on where you decide to go and in what country you are receiving the services from.

The average patient goes through two IVF cycles on average, bringing the total cost of IVF (including procedures and medications) between $40,000 and $60,000. (Single Care 2020)

IVF children are more frequently admitted to hospitals than non-IVF children. The post-neonatal hospital care cost of singleton IVF children was nearly two times that of singleton non-IVF children. (Human Reproduction 2007)

It is different from country to country. In Europe, many countries have economic support from the government for IVF treatments. When I was in the loop in Sweden, we had three IVF tries paid for by the government. You had to pay for all the medication yourself, but it was reduced a lot. Hormones are expensive. I recommend you look up the alternatives for your country. Countries have different laws and what is legal or not. For example, the donation of eggs and sperm is allowed in some countries but not in others.

JOURNALING

I strongly recommend journaling during your process. During heavy periods and with IVF treatments. I did journal, but I had difficulties writing down my feelings because it was too painful emotionally. When I started to write my diary, I only captured WHAT happened with no feelings at all. Admitting my feelings was too painful. Afterward, I realized that I did a detailed job of keeping track of all the treatments, but I did not journal or mention my thoughts and feelings that were spinning around my mind and through my body. I am convinced that it is most important to take care of feelings and thoughts because they affect your mind, body, and organs. With my knowledge, today, it was one big reason why I had so much trouble. *The Body Keeps the Score*, by Bessel Van Der Kolk, M.D., is a book I have read and highly recommend that you read it too.

I have summed up the three major points of this chapter that I never want you to forget! Here they are:

1. You must **work *with* your body**, treating it as working with your best friend, not against it. Treat it with compassion, love, respect, and trust that it does want you to be healthy, ultimately.

2. **Listen to your heart** and do not always feel pressured to follow what your head tells you or what sounds most realistic at the moment. Grace yourself with the space and time to think through all considerations from your heart.

3. **Stay knowledgeable** every step of the way. Knowledge leads to confidence and self-advocacy. Knowledge is power.

For me, it took a lot of years to accumulate all the knowledge I have. Feeling empowered is a natural byproduct of this accumulation. This also leads to a lot of reflections and questions like, did I really need a hysterectomy? Maybe there were other ways, but I just didn't have the knowledge at that time. In the future, I believe a hysterectomy will not be the first option for "getting rid of" all the pain. If I could go back in time, I would be curious if I could have avoided a hysterectomy. Today, there are many more options to try before moving to surgery as the solution. Check around and research all the different options that are available before you make your decisions.

Chapter 5
Self-Work

"Nothing is impossible. The word itself says 'I'm possible!'"

— Audrey Hepburn

This chapter is so important! I am excited for you to be launching into a section that is all about the "self." This chapter isn't necessarily more important than the others, but important in elevated ways. To start off, I am asking you to take an inventory of where you are right now, in your life, with yourself. I mean really, really take a look at yourself, and ask yourself questions like: How are you feeling? What is challenging you? What do you need to improve upon to experience this journey in the best way? Are your needs being met by your partner? Are you aware of any boundaries that you need to uphold more strongly?

I will share with you some of the battles and challenges I had with myself that are common for many women enduring gynecological problems. I will also share with you some of my deepest feelings that were tough to go through but at the same time, necessary to move forward and for my growth, recovery, and healing. I hope this chapter entices you in ways that will be helpful to you and your own unique situations.

SHAME & SELF-COMPASSION

During my journey, I felt a lot of shame. I was ashamed of having a body that did not function properly, like a car. Instead of leaking a ton of oil all the time, I was leaking heavy loads of blood and did not feel ok. I distinctly remember always sneaking around and having a tampon or pad ready at a moment's notice. It was traumatic to meet with friends to celebrate their pregnancy, to see a baby belly, or to see a stroller on the street. (Yes, traumatic. That is not too strong of a word to describe my reactions). I felt left alone and outside of the normal world that was happening around me. I had questions like: *Why doesn't my body work normally? What have I done wrong? What can I do to solve this? What have I missed?* This leads me to wonder what questions you are torturing yourself with. I wonder if you are searching, like I did, for anything that could take me out of my miserable state.

A woman feels bad, ashamed, and not normal when she has heavy periods or cramps, has to cancel events, or can't get pregnant. Self-esteem and self-worth go down the drain with every shower you must take to clean yourself up, and sometimes multiple showers in one day. All these things add to the pile of already overwhelming feelings of shame, low self-esteem, and little self-worth. This became so hard for your body, heart, and mind to carry.

To make things worse, sometimes in a situation when you at least expect it, these self-deprecating emotions show their ugly heads. It could be when you walk in at the waiting room for the IVF treatments. You look around and see some other couples there, and it hits you like a fist in the stomach that you are all there because of the same reasons: the women cannot get pregnant, and you feel like you are losers. That is how my mindset was. None of the people in those rooms have a body that works as it is supposed to. It feels like stepping into "the room of shame" where everybody knows why you are there. For me, I also recognized when some couples disappeared but we were still coming back.

I want you to know that you are NOT a loser. I ask you to throw the shame, low self-esteem, and low self-worth out of the window. I regret not doing this when I was there. I wish I had the tools, knowledge, and energy to have let it all go. I will tell you to focus only on why you are here, the specific reason: You long to create a new life. A new miracle. A precious gift of a baby! Refocus on the silver linings. It is great that you have the courage to step into that waiting room! Hug yourself or do a happy dance! Without the tests, you would not know what your body is struggling with. Maybe you find out that something is broken, or maybe the doctors can't find anything wrong. Whatever it is, you will be able to deal with it. You will be able to move past it. You will get to the other side. When you have heavy periods or trouble getting pregnant, you are preparing yourself with the courage to act so you can continue to get help and support. No one else knows how it is to be you. Each and every woman has their own journey and always remember the following:

- Only YOU know what a heavy period for you is.
- Only YOU know how much pain is too much.
- Only YOU know how devastating it feels not to get pregnant normally.
- Only YOU can tell yourself to remember: How can anybody support and help you if you don't speak up to others about what you are dealing with and what your needs are?

You know your body the best. You are the one to take care of it and do all you can to support yourself. There can be many reasons why your periods are so heavy, why your painful periods keep repeating themselves, or what "trick" there is in store for you to get pregnant. So much is involved to unravel. There is so much that has to be 100% aligned: nutrition, stress, age, environment, sleep, and even movement. In this book, I hope you get a lot of insights and support to feel better and to really get to know what to do more or less or where to turn.

Remember, too, that not being able to get pregnant is a lot like experiencing many other traumas. It is traumatic. To support yourself when experiencing this kind of trauma is to mindfully stay open and to stay connected to a new mantra: "I can't get pregnant." Please don't blame yourself or your body. Try to see it like you are dealing with a mystery, the unknown and maintain your curious state for as long as possible. Stay curious! I know it can be rough and too much to handle at times. I have been there, drowning in too much pain while being exhausted. I had so much shit to deal with! That time in my life felt like a giant roller-coaster. It was hard to stay present at times. When you have your horrendous periods and then IVF treatments, there are a lot of hormones flying around that just spice things up even more!

When the repeating cycles of shame or lowness come back, ask yourself what could support or help you in that moment. Maybe you can create your own emergency toolbox. Use a shoe box and decorate it if you like. Put things in it that you know can cheer you up. Maybe some chocolate, a candle, a fancy teabag, soft socks, some kind notes to yourself, a pad of paper for you to write to yourself, notes from loved ones of encouragement, or even a relaxing magazine. This can be your "go-to box" when you need it. Your own fantasy is the limit. When you need some self-care, grab the box, cuddle up in your bed or couch, and start feeling better when you open the box. It is of critical importance to do this kind of self-care and self-work. Please take good care of yourself. Embrace the many ideas in this book. There are a lot more out there too, but this is a start!

SURVIVOR MODE

Maybe you experience the same feeling that I experienced in what I now refer to as "Survivor Mode." These are the days and times that go on, and you are stuck. You don't move forward. You stay still in the same spot. It feels like you just go on with your days in survival mode. You may feel frozen, numb, or even disassociated from the real world a bit. But we don't just want to survive. We want to live and enjoy life and thrive. We deserve to get to the other side.

There, in survival mode though, it can feel dark and cold, and you have a hard time finding the light and way out. Please put this label on this time. Call it and name it "Survival Mode." Tell your partner when you are in this mode. Naming it takes some of the power away. Naming it helps you to push it away. Naming it reminds you that there are other names out there too, like resilience, perseverance, courage, faith, love, and strength. And remember, it hurts. It all hurts but there will be a time that comes where you don't feel numb anymore. In the meantime, it's okay to feel broken and to accept any help you need.

In the process of healing from heavy periods/ trying to get pregnant, here are some additional questions we must ask ourselves. Questioning helps you to understand yourself, become aware of your needs more, and receive clarity:

- What is most important?
- Do I need to put in all the extra hours at work?
- Where is the time for me and my life, and what do I long for?

- How can I accelerate the process of healing from heavy periods and also getting pregnant?
- If I cannot, how do I deal with it?
- Is there any chance I can find a different job that offers more time off, less work, benefits, working from home, or whatever that will better serve me and my partner?

I felt that I had to go to work no matter what. I pushed myself way too hard, and I paid the price with my sanity and with my health. I think the newer generations are much better at taking care of themselves and putting their needs first, but if you don't do that and feel pressure from work/yourself/parents/partner, it is time to reset and refocus on yourself. If you are working, I hope your employer understands what you are going through. I was open and told my closest team and boss what was going on. When people we are with daily know and are somehow involved, they often have a more open mind and understanding. If you don't say anything, it will be hard to explain sometimes why you must change your schedule or arrive late more often.

Unfortunately, not all work/family/friends are understanding and supportive. If your work does not understand you and your needs, it would help to look for another position elsewhere if at all possible. If your family/friends do not understand or support you, try to keep them at a distance or find ways not to listen or get upset. Reach out to your inner circle of besties, your pillar people, and your other support team members, as identified in chapter 8.

People react in all different ways to what you are going through. They react. They project. They can even be hurtful in other ways. Most of my closest friends and family wanted to understand and support me, but I had other experiences, too. I got a letter from a friend who did not understand and asked me to pull myself together! Can you even believe it? She wrote angry and mean things to me. She was hurt and felt rejected in immature ways. She could not accept the fact that I was focusing on other things in my life that were way different from what we used to focus on together. It can be sad and hard, but you have to let them go and live your own lives.

If you have a job and are earning money, you are most likely living a lifestyle up to your standards. Today, there is still a lot of pressure to live a "perfect life with a perfect job and a perfect body." All the expectations from society put undue pressure on us. Ask yourself some tough questions, like do you need to have it all? Ask yourself, how does my life need to change to allow the resources for me to move forward with dealing with heavy periods/getting pregnant?

I encourage you to look for options to put yourself and your health and what you are longing for as your first priority. You don't have to do everything. You don't have to bring home the bacon, cook the bacon, and above all, eat the bacon. Make a list of what is important for you and what is not so important, and see if you can make any changes. It might be easier or clearer to see what you can do when you write things down in black and white.

When I entered the car after surgery once, I had pain, felt ugly and awful, and didn't see a meaning in life anymore. The radio was playing a song. It was "Stronger" by Kelly Clarkson. I will never forget this song, to this day. I find myself humming it out loud or even hearing it in my head at odd times. The song lyrics were, "What doesn't kill you makes you stronger. Stand a little taller..." and it goes on with "Think you've had the last laugh? Bet you think that everything good is gone." Kelly Clarkson really knew what she was talking about! At that exact moment in time, when I got in the car, I felt everything in that song. It went through my veins. It sank into my heart. It spoke to me like a prayer coming directly to me, down from heaven. "All the good is gone. How can I laugh again?" The most important line for me was, "What doesn't kill you makes you stronger," and this is true. For every hard time, you grow taller. It does not feel like that at the moment, but somehow, we move on and find a way to a lighter place where we can laugh and enjoy ourselves again. This is called getting to the other side. You will get there.

GOOD GIRL SYNDROME

I had (and sometimes rarely still have) good girl syndrome. By good girl syndrome, I mean we want everything to be good; we are stuck as people-pleasers, which really falls into the personality type of "fawn." Fawning is also called a "please and appease" response and is associated with chronic people-pleasing and codependency habits. When in fawn mode, you seek safety by always wanting things to be "harmonious"; therefore, you want to always meet the wishes and demands of others. As women, when we are in this mode for years, we lose sight of our own needs. It is not so hard to naturally become a good girl. Many of our moms grew up that way, and we followed suit. As they say in the movie *Barbie*, it is literally impossible to be a woman because:

- You are beautiful and smart, yet you don't think you are good enough.
- A woman should be thin but not too thin.
- A woman should always work, support, and help others but not take too much space.
- A woman should act like a superwoman and,
- Always be prepared to support others while ignoring herself.

Many of us have the inner critics (ego mindset) that does not always help either. The inner critic is in our brain. You must become aware of your inner critic. That's the voice that always criticizes what you do or do not do. I suggest you start to fight back. I found a fun way to work with my inner critic, and maybe it will suit you too. I looked for a dog that could represent my inner critic. I can see her in my imagination. Her body shape, color, and how she acts. You can give her/him a name. When she (your inner critic, ego) starts shit-talking to you, tell her to shut up! Tell her to lie down and behave. Talk back to her to tame her evil, nasty, and negative crap chatter. I hope this tool helps you. On the flip side, you can also have another dog/cat that is nice and always supports you. See the shape and color and give a name. That dog/cat is the one that tells you good stuff and tells you to listen to your heart. Start paying more attention to the lovely dog as a way to work on building up your self-esteem. You are worthy. You are good enough.

SELF-LOVE & HEARTFULNESS!

A great way to take care of yourself is to listen to your heart and be gentle to yourself while living fully in the present moment. In the morning, I recommend grounding yourself to be better prepared for your day. You connect to your heart and check in with yourself. Think about your day and what you will be doing. Set up boundaries to protect yourself during your upcoming day in the areas that you feel more fragile with, like your energy, time, stressors, or in dealing with negative people. At the end of the book, there will be a description of what you can do to ground yourself.

Another way to take care of yourself is to go out in nature. It does not mean you need to go to a forest or on a hike. It can just be a walk in the park where you can enjoy the trees and flowers. If possible, take off your shoes and feel the grass under your feet.

This is a form of grounding where research has been conducted. Your feet absorb the energy from the life and ground below you. Back to basics is the best way to self-care.

Treat yourself as well as you treat your best friend. You have probably heard that before, but do you actually do that? Are you kind, loving, and gentle to yourself?

Think of things that make you happy or make you feel good. It can be the smallest things in life that really brighten up your day and in the long-term make your life a better place when you notice them and enjoy them all: a good cup of coffee, a bath in the evening, someone saying something kind to you, birds singing, a phone call from a friend, a pedicure, a massage. Only you know what makes your heart smile. Try to observe what brings a smile to your face or in your heart and be grateful for it.

Become a memory collector during this time. When we collect the great moments in life, we are rich in something that no one can take away from us. Try to do something each day that is gentle, kind, or fun. If you are a bit like me, let your inner child play. I love doing crazy things. People may think many different things about me because of this, but more importantly is that I enjoy my life in some capacity every day, as long as it does not hurt anyone! When you hear a great song in the store, start to move your body and take a few dance steps! I promise it makes you feel good.

Regarding my silly and playful side, I have been known to buy water balloons to have a water balloon fight on a warm day. I love April Fool's Day and take every opportunity to sing, dance, or whatever the joy. Music, dancing, and singing in the kitchen or bathroom can make you happy! Don't be shy. Life is too short. Stop walking for a short bit when you feel the sun coming out and let it shine on your face. Close your eyes and take a deep breath. It only takes a few seconds, and it changes a lot. Something that little puts a smile on my face. Start to do things that make you happy. Start today.

During your journey with heavy periods, hormone treatments, or IVF, and trying to live a normal life, you think, how am I supposed to enjoy life when it is so difficult, painful, and bad some days? You must allow yourself to feel sad and low. That is part of the process, so we must accept those feelings. Host a pity party for yourself. Play sad music, have an ugly cry, and hit something (preferably a pillow or something soft, but hit hard; let it out). or whatever you need to release what needs to be released. Don't push it down. Do not keep the negative energy inside.

Then, try to be gentle and kind to yourself even in these moments. You do your best, and sometimes we need to let it out to be able to carry on. We are often taught that showing sadness or that you are exhausted, overwhelmed, and need a break is not a good thing. It relates to that you are weak and not good enough. We need to learn and accept all those feelings. They come with a human body, and we are only whole and our authentic selves if we allow all feelings. Feelings are necessary. Feel them. Release them. Move on. That is self-care.

GRATEFULNESS

When we can be grateful and feel grateful for things we have or experience, we will have a more joyful life. It can be the smallest things or moments. Just think for a moment of how magical it is that you woke up today! You sleep in a cozy bed, you are in a free country, you have friends (I assumed all these things). You have bad periods, and your body works as it should for the most part. Take a moment each day, in the morning or evening or when it suits you, to acknowledge something you are grateful for. For a while, I had a jar in my kitchen. Every day after dinner I took a note and wrote down something I was grateful for that day.

Maybe you would like to try it for yourself? After a week or month, I had a little ceremony with something good to eat and drink and read all my notes. It makes you realize how much you appreciate in life. If you prefer a notebook or journal that's up to you. When we apply gratefulness to our lives, it changes a lot, even if you are in a dark place and it feels like nothing can help you. Don't give up. Try some of these exercises, and you will slowly start moving to a better place where you don't think life is crap. I know it can be hard. You will stumble and fall, but we get back up and move forward. You are so much stronger than you think.

Also, please remember that our brain works better if it gets some movement in the body. We start a flow in our bodies, and that makes it easier for us to feel more grateful and in a better place. It all connects. Body, heart, mind, and soul. If you can add a small walk, some music you like, maybe do a few dance steps, or sing in the shower, those small movements will fill you with good feelings and start a change in your mind and body.

STRESS

What sabotages our bodies the most is stress. When we are stressed, we are in fight and flight mode. Fight and flight mode is important to have. We need those skills to survive. But we are not living on the savanna anymore, so we don't have to use it that much. When we are "on the go" all the time and never have time to get our stress levels or cortisol down, it affects our whole body and every organ, including our reproductive organs. We need to find tools or ways to calm down our system. You can do different things that help your body calm down, like breathing techniques, walking in nature, baking, painting, or doing what you know will help you to slow down. There's also our unconscious mind that is hard to reach, mostly during nighttime. If we help to relieve our stress, our para-sympathetic nervous system kicks in, which relaxes us, making a big difference in our bodies.

The most important is to use our tools in our daily lives. If you have stressful work and/or life, it is even more important to find those "waterholes" to recharge your body. The great thing is they make a huge difference in your body. Apply small breaks during your day. For example, practice the "Breathing Minute," as outlined in the exercises at the back of the book. If you apply the Breathing Minute 2-3 times during your day, you will notice a difference after a week or a little longer, depending on how stressed your body is.

Starting your day with some stretches works wonders for your body and mind. It helps your body start the flow in your meridians and lymphatic system so you have more energy and are calmer and balanced. It can be done in 5-15 minutes in the morning. Even if you are not a morning person, you will feel the difference when you start. It is not that hard to get up a few minutes earlier. If you are really tired, I recommend you start your daily routine in bed. When you wake up, start with 2-3 deep breaths. Breathe down to your belly and slowly release. Then stretch your body, move your legs from side to side, maybe do a little face massage, and think of something you are grateful for.

I also want to mention that anything you can do to have well-functioning, healthy lymphatics will be most beneficial. Healthy lymphatics are directly correlated with eliminating inflammation and enhancing the immune function of your uterus. These are two key components for creating a healing environment in your body. You will find some exercises you can start with at the end of the book! Try them for a week. That is not that long. See what differences they make with your body and mind. I think you will like it!

SLEEP

Our sleep is key to feeling good. With good sleep, we recover during the night, and the body will have cleaned, repaired, and updated what needs to be done. When we have a hard time falling asleep or wake up during the night and don't get our deep REM sleep, our bodies get out of balance. Not too long ago, we humans went to bed when it got dark and got up with the sun. Now we follow our own patterns and do not follow nature and its rhythm. We sabotage ourselves, our bodies, hormone levels, and wellbeing. If we were to change back to following nature's rhythm, we would benefit because we are definitely connected to nature. It has an impact on our anatomy, physiology, immune system, and hormones. You can feel tired and slow when you have been up late the night before, and your stomach is a bit weird, but even more so if you have been on a flight and are jetlagged. Many use their phone or iPads a lot, and the blue light fouls up our brains to think it is still daytime. When our brain thinks it is daytime, it does not start the production of melatonin. Melatonin helps us fall asleep, and cortisol helps us wake up. When one starts producing, the other reduces, and the other way around.

Melatonin has a big impact on our nervous system and hormones. Melatonin also supports the function of our ovaries and ovulation. Normally, melatonin starts to be produced around nine o'clock in the evening. But with blue light, it does not get the right input. Cortisol rises in the morning and increases your energy. Both melatonin and cortisol have anti-inflammatory characteristics and activate your immune system if they can work properly. They also influence many other hormones, which make them important for your wellbeing and the possibility of getting pregnant. Your sleep can have an impact on estrogen, progesterone, and ovulation and, therefore, impact the possibility of getting pregnant. Now you think, "Ooops! I don't sleep well. I'm screwed!!" DO NOT WORRY. There is a lot you can do to support your sleep and wellbeing and increase your hormone levels. Start with the following check on your evening routine:

- What time do you normally go to bed?
- What time do you get up?
- Do you sleep with your phone/iPad or other devices in bed?
- Do you bring food to bed?
- What do you do before you go to bed? Routines?

Some things that disturb the production of melatonin are stress, coffee, alcohol, and blue light from screens. Make a decision to fully support your sleep. This will automatically help to heal your body in places you need healing. You can do a lot and it does not have to be big changes. When you create conditions for your body to get a restful sleep, you support one of the biggest foundations in your body for health and happy hormones. When you start, be gentle with yourself and see what is doable right now. Take it step by step. We do not want to add more stress! What you can do to support better sleep:

- Try to go to bed at the same time. Preferably around 10 pm.
- Get up at the same time every day. If you get up around 7 am, you help the cortisol production to start your energy production.
- Have a cool temperature in your bedroom. It helps to get better sleep.
- Start your bedtime routine one hour before you go to bed by stopping blue screen time. Enjoy a bath, a cup

of tea, or a book. Turn down the lights to help your body transform into a night mood.

- Take a bath or shower before bed. Warm water helps start the production of melatonin.
- Do not keep phones or other blue screens in your bedroom. Keep them outside your bedroom. Buy a battery alarm clock or help yourself get up when your phone goes off outside your bedroom!
- You can take Magnesium and Glycine before bedtime. Magnesium supports your body and muscles to better sleep, and glycine supports your deep sleep. Glycine is an amino acid that is a building block for making proteins in your body, a critical element for rest.
- Do some deep breathing or meditation when you go to bed.
- Think of something you are grateful for that you experienced that day. It helps you fall asleep with a great feeling in your body and heart.

THOUGHTS & EMOTIONS

What the world and researchers haven't realized until quite recently is that our thoughts and feelings affect us much more than we think. How we feel and how we think about ourselves have a big impact on our wellbeing. We tend to think almost the same way we did yesterday. There is research that we don't change much of our thoughts from day to day. So, if we have started a dark pattern, it is not easy to get out of it. We need help to build a new way in our head, a new thought. That can be challenging. If we work with affirmations, we slowly start a new little path in our head, and it grows bigger until we have built a new highway of new thoughts and a new pattern. If we are depressed, stressed, and feel low, we benefit from help from someone outside to change our thought patterns.

I admit that I have been, and sometimes still am, good at saying bad things to myself in my mind. It sometimes is like there is one little elf, or more likely one devil and one angel, on each of my shoulders. One is nice, and the other is evil. My head is in between as they argue if I should do something or not. Have you ever heard those voices talking in your head? When we slow down and get still, we can hear all the noise in our heads. There is a constant talking. Why did I do that? What will they think? Maybe I should have got that? We mostly think we don't have this ongoing talk in our heads but observe for a few minutes how many thought that appears in your mind. Just by reading this you have a lot of thought and feelings jumping up. Right? How and what we think and feel affects our bodies and organs.

CHINESE MEDICINE

One area of interesting thoughts and philosophies that I have always been fascinated with is Chinese medicine. I have had interest in this for a while now. Of course, one of the most popular theories is about the Yin and Yang, more commonly known as the balance between the feminine and masculine. This is a fascinating area of energies to familiarize yourself with.

More importantly, we can learn much more about the body from Chinese medicine too! Understanding some aspects of this practiced medicine system is beneficial so we can better ourselves in even more ways. It teaches us that there are five main elements, also referred to as phases, that are associated with certain organs in our bodies. They are water, fire, earth, wood, and metal. They are connected to the cycles of creation, destruction, and transformation and are also associated with the heart, liver, lungs, spleen, and kidneys. The different organs are connected to feelings, such as the heart relates to joy.

Reflecting back, it's no wonder as to why I battled preeclampsia. For many years, I lived with all the feelings related to poor liver function: frustration, irritation, anger, and stress. Lungs are related to sorrow. Spleen with worry and kidney with fear. We can think whatever we want about Chinese medicine, but I am fascinated by it. I wish I had known about Chinese medicine when I was working dealing with getting rid of heavy periods and IVF because it would have positively affected my healing trajectory a lot.

Anger, frustration, and irritation are feelings that, according to Chinese medicine, cause stagnation in the liver and can lead to many different symptoms like painful periods, PMS, headache, dizziness, and fatigue. Worry is an annoying feeling that, according to Chinese medicine, can cause an energy knot in the lungs, heart, and spleen, which results in energy blockages or stagnation. This energy is called "Qi" (key), which means life force energy. In summation, a person's life force energy that travels through your meridians gets knotted up by their worry! This imbalance can cause late or painful periods, breast lumps, pale skin, shortness of breath, and chest pressure. Worry is meant to protect us, but we tend to worry too much about anything and everything in a chronic manner. We can't predict and control everything as it will lead to muscle tension, irritation, sleeplessness, fatigue, and concentration difficulties, but most of all, it takes away our possibility to be happy.

In Chinese medicine, fear has two categories: when you suddenly get scared and when you feel anxious. When anxiety lasts for a longer period, it affects the health of your organs and influences your hormones. This is a common reason why women in menopause get stronger menopause symptoms like hot flashes, dryness, and dizziness.

FEELINGS

We all have feelings and thoughts that affect us. I want you to reflect on how feelings and thoughts affect you and what you can do to support yourself. Describe what worries you or causes fear or anxiety. Write them down in your journal or start a worry journal. It helps when you put words to paper and off the mind. It gets it out of your head. Here are some starter questions:

- What feelings or thoughts dominate your thinking?
- Where in your body do you feel a particular emotion the most?
- Does this feeling or thought help you or serve you well? Or hurt you in some way?
- Does this feeling or thought help you in a specific situation?
- Does this feeling or thought limit you?
- What would you say to a friend who has these feelings or thoughts?
- What would help you move away from this feeling?
- Did I remember that a normal feeling or emotion only lasts ninety seconds and that after that, it will go away if I just let it? Feelings are not facts. It is me who chooses to ruminate or obsess over it. I need to choose otherwise. I need to redirect my inner dialogue.

You can also separate the worry, fear, frustration, etc., from what you have power over and what you don't have power over. This is a good one for your list as well: what do I really have control or power over in this situation and can I let it go? Maybe you can get additional help from the Serenity Prayer by Reinhold Niebuhr. Here is an excerpt:

Annika Östberg

God/Divine/Source (Insert your preference)
Grant me the serenity to accept the things I can't
    change,
The courage to change the things I can,
And the wisdom to know the difference.

We all carry many different feelings, and quite often, we carry them for way too long. Feelings can limit us, make us suffer, and create dark thoughts and destructive feelings that pull us down. With all this going on in an uncontrolled manner, we can feel desperate because of our situation. We can feel stuck and suffer. Much of this will not change for us unless we remember one key ingredient to our wellbeing. There is something much bigger and more powerful: LOVE. That's why we are here. Love creates love. Love creates life. In our daily lives, we easily forget how powerful our bodies and minds are. With self-love and love from others and our divine powers, we will endure. Our own body has the ability to reach into the deep caverns of love that we carry with us. Love will help to reunite us with our innate wisdom and intelligence.

Along with emotional feelings, please remember the simple things around our bodies" needs. They need fresh, clean water, light fresh air, and a connection to the Earth, just like a simple flower. You are a miracle, and you have the possibility to heal and recover far beyond your imagination with the access to and use of these ingredients. our bodies can heal and recover. Please believe this, especially if we treat it in a good way. Going back to the fundamental things like water, food, nature, and air is valuable. If not, we often take things like this for granted and still retain expectations of how our bodies are supposed to work. But if you do a simple inventory of the simple, daily things you are doing or not doing to your body, you will be surprised at how much you can improve. We can't simply order our bodies in terms of how they function. The only thing we can do is to create the best possible conditions for our bodies and minds to thrive and blossom. Remember that baby step by baby step. We have the power to change our way of living.

Each and every day in every situation, we have the possibility to choose how we want to feel and react. This is called living with intention. When you do not live with intention, you go through life in reaction mode. This soon becomes unmanageable and unhealthy. Here is a simple example of being intentional about how you handle something simple in life. One day, while I was at a café, the lady next to me spilled her coffee all over herself. I watched her closely as I really expected to hear some profanity or angry outbursts. Instead, she started laughing and in a most delightful way! She chose to laugh at herself instead of being angry and upset that she got coffee all over herself. Can you imagine how much less stress we all would be under if we chose to live more intentionally instead of in reaction mode?

Another example is Nelson Mandela, a well-known South African President and resistant leader. He was incarcerated for twenty-eight years. He suffered badly. They had him digging his own grave, and the guards peed on him. What do you think he decided to do? He chose how to feel and think about his situation. He chose not to hate the guards and not to react with violence. Instead of hate and anger, he chose love. Hate and anger would not have helped him or the guards. This is another testament to the power of love and self-love. One of his famous quotes is, "Do not judge me by my successes. Judge me by how many times I fell down and got back up again."

For me, when I was upset, angry, or ashamed with my body, with some treatments, or with my doctors, I didn't know that I could actually choose my reaction, my thoughts, and feelings. Instead, I just reacted automatically, and not in a good way. As a result, I soon became a victim and fell into victim mode unintentionally.

I ask you to take some time to really think about how you want to feel and react to situations while you are on this journey, that are hard and unfair. Do you want to be a victim of your thoughts and feelings? It is not easy to accept some things, like heavy periods or not getting pregnant, but if you chose more compassionate, positive feelings and thoughts, your body and organs won't be as affected or impacted nearly as negatively. Your body keeps the score. Wouldn't this new, healthier approach be awesome to practice and eventually master?

LOVE

Love that is born from your heart has incredible powers. In your heart, there is no space for negative or destructive feelings or thoughts when it is full of love and gratitude. These two beauties, love, and gratitude together, are often neglected or forgotten when you are on this incredulous journey. But you can't destroy love because it is not just one feeling. Love is a complicated emotion that is so much bigger than one human feeling. Love is deep, tender, complete, affection, connection, and devotion, to name a few. Love is all-encompassing. We tend to forget love. The love of ourselves. The love to our own body. We tend to have expectations on our bodies how it should work and when it does not follow our plan, when our bodies complain through symptoms, we tend to be disappointed with our bodies instead of treating then with care and love.

In most of our lives in today's world, the expectation is that everything is supposed to work fast and smooth, but this perception spreads to the overall opinion about our bodies. Most of us expect our bodies to function properly and to perform as required. This sets us all up for disappointment and emotional strife. When our bodies have symptoms that we don't like, I encourage you to start with self-compassion and with love as your first reactions. It can feel overwhelming at first because you are disappointed with your body and are probably used to being in this mood. But, as cheesy as it sounds, love conquers all. To start to love yourself, which includes your incredibly beautiful body, is to choose a much more positive way.

Only you can learn and know intimately how to take the best care of your own body. It does not have to be difficult, especially with new routines developed. At any time, you can take a deep breath and let your shoulders relax and jaw drop softly open. Think about your body. Send it love. Feel your heart beating and know that it loves you too. Don't take this for granted. To honor our bodies, our fantastic bodies, that carry us through life on this Earth each and every day, is huge. Promise your body that you will take good care of it, that you are happy and grateful for your body, that it is a miracle, and that you are on this journey together. Hand in hand, you can take the steps toward your goals. Support, nourish, and honor your body with great food, rest, movement, and joy, and your journey together will be spectacular. It all starts with self-love.

With self-love, you will be in better contact with your body and closer to your heart. That leads to less time with your thoughts, worry, and fear in your head and closer to your heart. The most important relationship in your life is the relationship you have with yourself. When you focus on self-love, your heart expands and pushes away negative thoughts and feelings. Sounds strange? Give yourself a real try. Understand that you ARE a miracle. You can heal, create, and survive so much with self-love. Witness how you feel after you tell yourself these affirmations. Here are some to start with:

- I am worthy.

- I deserve to be loved.
- I am good enough.
- I am enough.

Here are some other ways to feel and expand your self-love:

- **Accept yourself as you are and where you are.** Enjoy the moment because that's the only thing you can control. Be here and now. Even on the worst of days, you can find something that lights you up. It can be the smallest thing.
- **Forgive yourself and your mistakes.** Stop criticizing yourself for things you have done or did not do. Don't blame yourself. You did the best you could in that moment.
- **Celebrate every success.** Every little, small thing that you achieve is worth celebrating. We tend to celebrate too little in this world.
- **Be grateful.** Notice all the small things in your life that you take for granted: your bed, home, shower, flowers, birds singing, friends, a stranger's smile, that you have a body that works most of the time! Show gratefulness by saying thank you in your heart to every small thing that comes your way. Say thank you to all that have happened to you because it led to who and where you are today. Small steps of gratefulness will change your life.
- **Love & Heart Meditation.** Listen to meditations with a focus on self-love, self-awareness, or similar.

Take moments to feel your heart and love for yourself and

your body. Feel how your love expands and fills up your body. It can be hard at the start because you are not happy with your body, but be gentle and kind to yourself, and soon you will notice a shift. Whisper or say *"I love you"* in your head to yourself. *"I love you."* It can start a lot of feelings when you really pay attention and listen to your own words. Tears can appear or a small crack of a smile shows up. Start each day by saying *"I love you"* to yourself for some time and see what happens. Try to look yourself in your eyes in the mirror as you say, "I LOVE YOU!" When you mean it, it will bring up all different feelings. Embrace them. It may feel or sound silly, but it is powerful.

The mastery of self-love takes time and practice. Be patient. Make a starting agreement with yourself that says "I will love you. I will be more intentional with my behaviors and less reactive." Remove the control you think you have to have and remove the judgment that comes from your egocentric inner critic. Build this new self-love practice into your life until the love for yourself is undeniable, strong, and empowering.

Chapter 6
IVF: Invitro Fertilization

"There is no list of rules. There is one rule. The rule is: There are no rules. Happiness comes from living as you need to, as you want to."

— Shonda Rhimes

Do you know how long IVF treatments have existed? Maybe you do, but most likely not. Here is some quick history. The first baby born through IVF treatment was Louise Brown. She was born in 1978. In 2010, there were more than four million humans born from this technique. Sir Robert Edwards was the pioneer in the reproduction field, specializing in IVF fertilization. He tried to fertilize the eggs in a petri dish before implanting a two-and-a-half-day-old embryo. In 2010, he received a Nobel Prize in medicine for the development of in vitro fertilization. This method has helped millions of infertile couples worldwide to have children.

Today, Louise Brown is living a normal life. She is married and has two kids that were "made" normally. Her parents had tried for many years before they got this opportunity. In the news, when this was exposed to the public, the pope was concerned that this method could turn women into baby factories, and the Catholic church announced that artificial insemination, in vitro fertilization, and surrogate motherhood were immoral. However, all these methods have helped many people in their quest to have a baby. Today, there are about eight million IVF kids worldwide.

If you are considering IVF or have already started it, it is imperative that you have a heads-up that the IVF testing, procedures, and treatments do not necessarily stop when you get pregnant. You still may need hormones for a while to support your body. There are many tests and procedures that follow. You and your partner need to discuss what tests you want to do to check the baby's health. And WHAT you will do in different scenarios. If the baby is handicapped, for example, what do you think about that? What is your plan, and what do you both believe? As a couple, talking about how you feel and what you want if something is wrong is good.

There is so much more to consider and think about after you get pregnant, too. You may need to support your body differently, and I want you to know that. The 24/7 mindful self-care and attention do not stop when/if you get pregnant. You may need more rest or other things after the hormone treatment that you did not think of. You may have the same fluffy pink dream I used to have that pregnancy is so cute and perfect. Of course, it is cute and a miracle in the making, but it can be a bit more exhausting after an IVF treatment. If you have had a miscarriage before, like I did, you might be afraid to lose the child. Fear is no friend. Find ways to focus on the happy thoughts!

EMOTIONAL REFLECTION

During my journey with endometriosis, hormone treatments, and then in vitro, I often felt lost. One doctor recommends something, and the next time, another doctor wants to try something else. I felt like a Test Rabbit. Every doctor wanted to try something new and have success. It was all centered around them trying to have my body do and make the right thing. It was never how I felt and how my body and mind were connected. You listen to the doctors and follow their advice because you are desperate and don't know what to do. You are dealing with such a myriad of feelings. You feel depressed and sad and just want to find a solution. You want to feel better during your periods, or at least functional. Then, on top of it all, you are wishing for positive results from your IVF.

Of course, it is wonderful that the doctors tried to help me. I am grateful for that. But as time went by, as the years passed, I became even more in a depressed state. I started to numb myself. I combined heating pads on my abdomen with painkillers to help me deal with my emotional and physical pain. But it did not help, so I added alcohol. When you are in a life situation where you feel desperate for relief, you try different coping mechanisms. It is so easy when you are in the loop of treatment with doctor's visits, blood draws, etc.., that you have no time to think about other things or reflect.

During the IVF treatment, **everything** in your life fully centers around the treatment regime: doctor's visits, scheduling blood draws, juggling work schedules to be able to go to all required appointments, phone calls with new instructions, getting other injections in time, and taking any other medications. This whole lengthy regime swallows up your whole life and your partner's life too. It becomes really stressful. You hang on to the hope that it will be worth it because you will be rewarded with having a baby, but it was already months and most likely years ago when you started the process. It is common and normal to feel a little bit freaked out because you're doing a lot to your body while also dealing with the disappointment that your body did not work as it was supposed to do.

HORMONE TREATMENTS

Doses of hormone treatments are so strong and powerful. I felt like the doses I was administered were really made for horses, not for a little woman! I don't know how much research there has been done on the doses. Probably a lot, but my body is still working after 16 years to recover from all the treatments. IVF hormone treatments are way too hard on our bodies. They have a big impact on your emotions and mental stability. You are playing like "GOD" with your body, really trying to make things happen in your body in an unnatural way. How much is too much? Just look at bodybuilders that use hormones to build up their bodies. They get big muscles fast and often, also have a bad temper, and their body can never recover. When they stop exercising and taking hormones, their body gets different issues. You are not a bodybuilder, and your medical team will keep you under good supervision, and there is no experimenting. But in some way, you experiment with your body.

My advice for you is to do as much research as possible on the recommended treatments you are being guided on. If I knew what I know today, I would have tried alternative methods much earlier. If I knew what I know today, I would have gone another path. I was a bit into it, but people around me were of another opinion. What If I had known then and truly believed as I do now that our bodies are miracles and can heal from much more than we think? I wonder what it would have been like. I want you to really listen to your own body and mind.

- What is the best solution for you?
- What would your body benefit from most?
- How much are you ready to invest in the treatments?
- Are you more traditional, or do you prefer alternatives? Either way, this is about your body, and I ask you to treat it gently and with love. You are so much stronger and wiser than you think!

Whatever you choose as your course of treatment, it is important to take care of yourself with healthy food and a healthy lifestyle with a balance between activity and rest. Spend some moments to think about the questions and check with your body and heart on what resonates with you the most. I have gotten great results working with my clients with energy medicine. One young woman had heavy bleeding and cramps that led to some days home from school. The period normally lasted for a whole week, seven days, or a bit more. After working with her for less than ten months, her bleeding was down to five days. They were still quite heavy, but she was in much less pain. That is a huge difference. She could act normally and do activities and sports even during her period.

I am blown away by how energy can work in our bodies, the removal of energy blockages, and the starting of energy flows. She also was eating healthy and tried to live a balanced life between activity and rest. Get enough sleep and try to keep stress levels low. In summary, it made way for her success! Our bodies are miracles if we let them do the work. Never forget this. Never forget that your body does want to be healthy. It wants balance. It desires to be healthy. Put your positive mindset to work to support what your body is also craving.

There could be many different reasons why a pregnancy does not occur. For a man, it could be that the sperms are slow or there are too few. For a woman, it could be that the fluid is not right in the cervix or the uterus, and the embryo can't attach. Maybe there is something not quite right with the eggs. The list can go on and on. Also, it may not just be one reason behind the challenges. There could be one thing or many things preventing a pregnancy. Working closely with your doctors to assist you in discovering exactly what your challenges are is a critical step in your ability to make decisions on how to best move forward in your life. Do a lot of research on any subject that you feel a deep dive would be valuable. Below is a list of common reasons why it may be difficult to get pregnant.

CHECKLIST & REASONS WHY PREGNANCY IS DIFFICULT

Age – A woman's fertility slows down sometimes after 30. Your hormone levels change, and egg quality is reduced. The risk of miscarriage rises with age as well, unfortunately.

Sperm—Quality and quantity are two of the most critical aspects of healthy sperm. There must be enough sperm, and the quality and shape of the sperm are important. Learn as much as you both can about this area.

Eggs – The quality of the eggs is a high priority. When you are about twenty-five years old, you have about 75% of your eggs with normal chromosomes. As you age, this percentage decreases. When you are around thirty-five years old, you will have approximately 50% of your eggs with normal, healthy chromosomes. Then, at age 40, this number reduces to 10-15% on average. You can see how the number goes down, but you can see that even at age 35 years old like I was, you still have a 50% chance of normalcy! I got so sick and tired of hearing "Tick Tock, Tick Tock" in my brain as well as from other people.

Tubes –Do they have free, unblocked passages, for example? What is their overall health like?

Uterus – Is it unhealthy? What about the form and position?

Ovaries – There are many aspects to the ovaries: egg production, releasing eggs, damage to any of the ovaries or eggs, and many more. Research and remember, Knowledge is Power.

Cervical fluid – Is the fluid healthy? Be sure to ask your medical team about this aspect and understand it in full.

STDs – If you have any, including chlamydia, and they are left untreated, there can be impacts that you do not want. Ensure that this is fully checked out and managed.

Obesity – Research indicates that it can make pregnancy more difficult. I am not sure of all the reasons, but you can research this aspect further if obesity is, for some reason, a concern.

Underweight – Research indicates that this, too, can make pregnancy more difficult.

Alcohol and drugs – These are definitely areas of concern; their use or addictions have a huge impact. Rely upon your doctors to guide you in the best way regarding any of these concerns for you or your partner/sperm donor.

Cysts, Endo, or PCOS – These are all indicative of influencing the ability to get pregnant. Stay on top of this if you are diagnosed and educate yourself thoroughly.

Stress is evil if it is too much! Stress levels affect the whole body, all organs, and your emotional and nervous system states. Understand what aspects of your life bring you undue stress and what triggers it. Be sure to offset it with exercise, good whole-food nutrition, and sleep.

Sperm – For some men, it is out of the question to check the quality of their sperm because of their ego. Yes, simply put, it is a sensitive topic. It can even be harder to talk about and the feelings around it. I hope this is not the case for you, and if it is, please seek help and guidance from some professionals on how to best work around this challenge. There are some ways to boost the quality, and your partner may just need some awareness and education to make the process comfortable. Here are ten science-backed ways to boost sperm count and increase fertility in men:

- Take D-aspartic acid supplements
- Exercise regularly
- Get enough vitamin C
- Relax and minimize stress
- Get enough vitamin D
- Try Ashwagandha
- Take frequent supplements
- Get enough zinc
- Joy! Have fun Either by yourself or together
- Be wary of too much heat in the sperm area (For example, car seat heat, hot tubs, heating pads)
- Eat healthy and mindfully

As you see, the list of reasons not to get pregnant is. There can be other reasons too that I haven't mentioned. These are some of the most common reasons. If you suspect any of these are possibilities, I suggest you do research. Do not only use Google, as this can lead to you getting scared and hypochondriac feelings and make you think you suffer from a lot. Believe me, I know from experience! It is much better to find a person with knowledge that can inform you accurately. If you don't think your ob-gyn can answer your questions, seek a second opinion. You can find different ways to find information, but you must make up your own mind and have confidence in what you learn, observe, and find out. Also, full disclosure to your partner. Transparency and full honesty will serve both of you well on this journey.

After trying to get pregnant naturally with no success, it can be a good idea to research if something is not as it is supposed to be, especially researching in detail the results of any tests or procedures you have decided to endure. You have probably already charted your cycle. Maybe you have been keeping track of your ovulation as well. If not, that is a great way to track when you have ovulation and the best time to get pregnant. You can buy those tests in most pharmacies. They work the same way as a pregnancy test. You pee on a little test strip, and it will tell you if now a good time is. You can also follow your cycle with a thermometer. Your body temperature changes with the cycle. The more you know about your body, the better.

TEST RABBIT

Every country has a different approach to IVF, but on the first visit to an IVF clinic, you have to answer a lot of questions; they take a blood draw and want sperm to be checked at a minimum. You will receive information about the process, and you have probably done a lot of research by yourself online already. The direction and steps the doctor recommends to you depend on what they will find. Surprisingly, quite often, they find that nothing is wrong with you. This may come as a huge surprise to you, too, accompanied by some angst and frustration. This is something that I understand fully. For so long, we have battled so much, and we are convinced that there is something wrong and that it must be obvious to the medical community. But, if nothing is found from this first, preliminary round of tests, we feel let down. It is paradoxical because why would we want to find something wrong with our bodies? Because we cannot get pregnant!

However, they may find something is wrong, like with the passageways in the tubes. Maybe the sample from the uterus shows something. Maybe the sperm is not quite what it needs to be. But again, remember that many times, nothing abnormal is found. Let me just mention again that this can come as a surprise and can make you feel disappointed because there can be some relief when a person does find out "what is wrong." Regardless, this is the time you should really consider alternative treatments, leveling up how you take care of yourself and what plan B, C, or D may be.

If something abnormal is found, and you can be treated for it, you may end up at an IVF clinic at your next appointment if this is an avenue you want to take. With an IVF treatment process, you probably start with a low-hormone treatment to support your cycle. If the low hormone treatment, in combination with you and your partner having sex, doesn't result in you getting pregnant, after many tries, you will then need to move to a next step. Keep in mind that the medical process differs from country to country.

IVF TREATMENT

I will share my journey, which is still relevant to most treatments. To start up the treatment, we "turned off" my body as a way to shut down the system. I did that through a nose spray! Isn't that weird? After only a few days of spraying, I started to notice symptoms of menopause, like being sweaty with hot flashes, tired, headachy, accompanied with sleep problems. I know it sounds horrible, and to be honest, it is. But after all the years of bleeding, pain, and everything else, I was a trooper!

The nose spray is developed to shut down your body and to have you go into menopause. It is easier to control the rebuilding of your cycle back to the beginning when you are in a menopausal state. Some women do not feel it much. I didn't feel that much the first time, but it got worse each time with heavy symptoms. Mostly, I had trouble with my dry nose and sinus at each treatment. Your doctor will check your status with a blood draw. The results will tell you if your body is in shutdown mode, also referred to as being in menopause. The levels of some hormones must be at a specific level. I will not go into all the different hormones and the numbers they are supposed to have in the different phases because there is so much data. Your medical community will provide all these details.

Keep the focus on the treatment procedure. Otherwise, you will be overwhelmed. At this stage, the hormones and numbers are not as important. When your body is in menopause mode, it is time to start building up the body to make the best, healthiest home for a pregnancy. That is when you start with hormone injections to build up the mucous membrane. To have the right physiological balance, you take the nose spray at the same time as you inject hormones, like stepping on the gas and brake pedal at the same time. You are monitored and managed regularly with a blood draw. There will be quite many blood draws, always in the mornings. It can be a bit tricky to fit in with your work schedule. The amount of hormone fluid that you need to inject can change depending on how you develop.

After each blood draw, you talk to a nurse in the afternoon to adjust the injections. When you have reached the right level, it is time to check the mucous membrane with an ultrasound. The doctor tells you if the mucous membrane is thick enough and if it looks good. They also check that you have eggs. Preferably, you have one or two eggs. If there is a thumbs up, it is time for the release the egg shot. You get a specific time when you must take the shot and then it is time to have sex. They will tell you that it would be good if you perform at least two – three times in the coming twenty-four hours. Whoop whoop! Just what you are longing for!! I hope you feel that way. I felt a bit bruised after the treatment and sensitive, but we were so ready to be intimate. Then you wait for some weeks, around twenty-one days, before you can do a pregnancy test. If you do it too early you can get a false positive test due to all the hormones. Better to wait patiently. If you got a negative result, there is next level.

If the above method is not successful, then it is time to increase the hormones to be able to harvest eggs and perform the fertilization with egg and sperm outside of the uterus. When the plan is to harvest eggs, they want you to have as many eggs as possible. Last time for me, it was like having bunches of grapes hanging off my fallopian tubes each side. It got sensitive and painful. I could only walk on my tiptoes and no heels on my shoes. Every step I took was awkward. My belly was swollen, and I could not walk far. My husband had to go grocery shopping and I felt a bit like a slow moving and stranded whale. When we harvested, I had eighteen eggs in total from both sides.

The procedure is the same. You start with nose spray and check with blood draw that your body is "turned off." Then you add hormones, with a bit more power than if you want a normal cycle. When you have reached the right level, it is time to check the mucous membrane and eggs with an ultrasound. If everything looks good, you get a specific time to take the release shot. It is important that you are right on time because you get an appointment to harvest the eggs at the best time.

At the clinic you have to dress in a surgery gown. You get a needle inserted on top of your hand as an IV and a pill to calm you down if you like. The "harvest room" looks like a surgery room with a gynocology chair. When you all are in place, the ob-gyn doctor and nurses start the process. You get some painkiller through your IV drip and then it is time to start the harvest. With a tool, the doctor enters through your vagina, goes up through your vaginal wall, punctures your vaginal wall to get into the ovary. Unfortunately, this is something that you can feel. You are not put to sleep, but you will get a pain killer. There the harvest starts. A nurse collects and counts the eggs. One nurse checks you, so you are alright and if you need more painkiller. When one side is finished, they collect from the other side. Your partner is allowed to support you and stand beside you and hold your hand if you like during this harvest process. It is not pleasant.

When all eggs are harvested, you get help to go back to the room where the nurse helped you prepare. You get some rest and something to eat. You need to go to the restroom so they know you are alright and can pee before you are allowed to go home. Before you leave, your partner needs to have his sperm harvested. Sometimes he needs to perform before you are able to get up from your bed. They have a room with some magazines that are supposed to help the process. While I was resting, it was our turn to harvest sperms. My husband went away to do his part. At least the men don't have to have anesthesia, needles, and surgery in the body to harvest the sperms. In the lab, the technicians follow the process to bring the eggs and sperms together for fertilization. After all that happens, you go home. The partner can go back to work, but for the woman, it is best to lay down and rest, spending time on the couch resting and with some painkiller. Maybe you need an additional day to recovery. If so, take it!

After a day or two you get a call when they tell you how many embryos that they got and how many that look perfect. They must be prefect to be accepted. To be perfect, they have to develop right number of cells and have perfect shape and size. You get a time to come back to the clinic to "transfer an embryo" back. When you transfer an embryo back to the uterus you get the same gown and socks as used for the surgery. You do not need any painkiller. Some doctors recommend that it is good if you have a quite full bladder. In the surgery room they check your name carefully. Then with a small hose, that they gently put all the way up into your uterus, they transfer the embryo back. They normally show you on a screen where it is. Then you just hope it will attach and stay there. In Europe, they normally only transfer one embryo.

In the United States, and in some other countries, they transfer more embryos. You have the same possibility to get pregnant with both options, but if many embryos attach successfully to your uterus, you get the option to reduce some because there is much risk with every additional embryo. There is an increase in the risk of a miscarriage with more than one embryo. If you have more embryos, then the one you transferred back that look perfect, you can freeze them for potential future use for yourself or you may possibly consider making them available for science. I harvested eggs two times. I stored a frozen embryo one time and used fresh ones two times.

After the embryo is back in the uterus, you often get hormone pills to put in the vagina. It can be up to three times a day. It is recommended to lay down for a bit after the pills are in place so they don't slip out right away. It is imperative that you lay down! You do not want gravity to make a play here to make it seep out! I wish science was a lot further along with this! It is also a good idea to have a small pad because it gets sticky. Sometimes you support with some hormone shots or pills as well the days after embryo returns.

It is different in different countries how much support you get from the government. In Sweden, for example, I think you get good support economically from the government. In other countries, it is probably a combination of your health insurance and your own out of pocket funding for these types of services. The IVF treatment costs a lot of money, time, patience, emotions, social life, etc. You invest a lot and hope for a miracle. It is a bit of a lottery. IVF is a gift, but it's not för everyone.

Chapter 7
Holistic & Alternative Treatments

"Other women who are killing it should motivate you, thrill you, challenge you and inspire you."

— Taylor Swift

Being fertility challenged is an arduous journey. The stigma alone is beyond challenging to deal with, let alone having the courage to try alternative treatments beyond the traditional. When you are in the thickness of despair, you become much more open to trying things that you wouldn't normally consider and hoping that all you combine to create your IVF arsenal will be enough. Below are such offerings that complement the combination of both east and western ways. Above all else, remember that you are on your own, individual treatment journey and that you are empowered to make your own choices around your assisted reproduction approach.

ACUPUNCTURE

I really don't like needles. In fact, I detest them. I'd like to say good bye to them all together for the rest of my life, but I came to that point as I mention above, where I was open to doing anything to get pregnant. I also was beyond dealing with the miserable state of constant bleedings. This malady, coupled with the stress, sleep deprivation and sneaky episodes of depression will make any woman consider alternate methods.

If you do some research, you will discover that acupuncture has been around for over 3,000 years. Something like this can only be around for that long if it has huge benefits! It basically stimulates points on our bodies that are "pathways" to our 2,000 meridians of energy flow. The needles open up these critical pathways that have otherwise been disrupted or blocked. Blood flow, stress reduction, balancing your endocrine system and stimulating your ovaries are just a few of the benefits you will discover in your research. Don't forget your partner either, as acupuncture treatments for them can positively correlate to increases and higher quality semen!

I heard of a famous certified, professional, and licensed acupuncturist woman in Sweden, that had helped one hundred infertile couples successfully get pregnant. So, I made an appointment with her. We only focused on strengthening the uterus so it could be able to carry a baby. After many years of heavy periods, hormone treatments and stress etc. my body was worn out and my uterus weak and soft. I can't recall how many treatments I had with her, but I think it was once a week for the last two months before the last IVF treatment. It worked! Acupuncture was immensely helpful in helping my uterus get strong enough to carry a baby, and for me, it was two babies that my amazing uterus was able to successfully carry! In retrospect, I summed it up that the combination of acupuncture, with all the other holistic methods I employed, was the secret sauce.

CHINESE MEDICINE TEA

I saw a Chinese doctor that checked my tongue, eyes, pulse, and other vitals and then gave me a special medicinal herbal tea to drink to support my body. They depend a lot on different herbs and will recommend that you use them to support your systems. They focus a lot on your whole body and not just one system because everything is connected. Chinese medicine focuses on how to help support your body to heal, Chinese medicine mostly concentrates on preventing illness but is also a great way to help your body. Different teas can that they recommend to drink regularly will result in many healing benefits.

MASSAGE

Massage is one hour of heaven on earth! I really enjoy a massage and it helps my body and mind to relax and to feel softer and smoother. I enjoyed many massages, especially in between the IVF treatments or in the beginning. When you have transferred an embryo back, you should not have a massage because the energies created and triggered in your body from the massage can affect you. During pregnancy, it is better to get the special pregnancy massage where the professional will know what trigger points not to touch that will gamble with your pregnancy, because otherwise it can start processes in your body so you might lose the child. This is critical to know. Let me be clear. Having a massage is not dangerous if the person working on you knows how to give you a "pregnancy" massage.

PEDICURE OR MANICURE

To pamper yourself, get a wonderfully relaxing pedicure or manicure. They are great ways to feel better. Another professional person takes care of you for an hour. They massage your hands or feet and make them look great and cleaned up beautifully. This can be a great self-care to brighten up your day! Maybe you even want to schedule this on a regular basis or just now and then. If you have never tried, maybe now is the time, especially if you take a buddy with you. It is just one more way to pamper yourself and feel better. Let me caution you by telling you not to allow the person who is giving you a pedicure to massage your feet or lower legs. I say this because I am a firm believer in our energy meridians, and we do not want to trigger these points! Massage to your feet or your lower legs can replicate foot reflexology.

FOOT REFLEXOLOGY

I had several foot reflexology treatments before I endured IVF to prepare my body to support my body before a new IVF treatment. Let me stress again that this was done **before my IVF, not during pregnancies.** Simply put, this works because, on your feet, you have acupressure points that are connected to your body parts and organs through nerves and energy flows. By stimulating these points, you activate the part of your body that is connected to this point on your foot. A foot reflex treatment is a great way to stimulate and help your organs relax, recover, and reload. It is mostly enjoyable, but for some people, some parts can be painful. If they are, this is the way that you know those points need attention and support. Be careful with who you go to. Check out that they have a great education and are certified/licensed and experienced.

MINDFULNESS & MEDITATION

Mindfulness is a wonderful tool to help you reduce stress and be more here and now, in the moment. It helps you recognize tension in your body, reduces it, and lets it go. Mindfulness clears your head and helps you get more focused in your daily life as well. You can find many great mindfulness meditations on YouTube. I really enjoy the short, ten-to-fifteen-minute videos that are actually meant for children. This is another example of my playfulness. I love to have a meditation where you are guided to a secret tree house or fairy garden! Check it out and see what you like. You can find longer and shorter meditations as well. If meditation is new to you, please don't be afraid and try to remove any skepticism. Easing and resting your mind in any way is so good for your overall wellbeing. Think of it as resting your mind. Meditations can help you fall asleep, calm your nervous system, and support you through your worry and anxiety, but they also provide lovely affirmations to help boost your mind with joy, happiness, and gratitude. Please give this a try. After a while, you will ache for this time as you know how beneficial it is. Here are some short facts about how mindfulness and meditation affect your brain:

- Reduces anxiety, depression, and rumination
- Improves decision-making
- Improves motivation and mood regulation
- Improves memory and learning
- Increases compassion & empathy

Here are some facts on how mindfulness & meditation helps your body:

- Reduces stress

- Improves immune response
- Decrease chronic pain and fatigue
- Increases nutrient uptake
- Increases fat-burning capabilities
- Reduces cellular aging
- Supports positive changes in gene expression

By applying mindfulness and meditation methods to your daily regime, you see and feel the benefits quite fast. It does not have to be sitting for one hour focusing on your breath, either. Start slowly and gently. Maybe set a timer for five minutes. Then you sit down comfortably and close your eyes. A great start is to take some deep breaths, but you can choose what suits you. Maybe focus on a candle or on your feet when you walk slowly. One great tool is "box breathing." You inhale, hold your breath, exhale, and then hold your breath, all in increments of four seconds. I see a shoe box in my imagination and breathe in as I follow one side up; along the long side, I hold my breath; down the short side, I exhale; and along the bottom side, I hold my breath. If you trace the box when you follow your breathing, you let all other thoughts fade. This is a tool the military uses to help soldiers calm down in stressful moments. Your blood pressure alone decreases as your parasympathetic nervous system is summoned by breathing. But it is great in our daily life as well! You don't have to be a Navy SEAL to practice this technique.

Don't blame yourself when your thoughts drift away because they will! You are only human, and we are supposed to use our minds a lot. Instead, every time öhen you drift away with your thoughts and you notice them, be kind and gentle to yourself. Say in your mind:" Ooops! Here we go again!" and take back your focus on your breathing. For each and every time you notice, you become more aware. Be grateful that you noticed. For every time you take your focus back to your breath throughout your day, you get closer to staying more focused and achieve more clarity, even in your daily life outside of the meditation.

YOGA

Yoga can be a great tool to support your body and mind. There are many different yoga styles, and you must try them out to see what your favorite is. There are as many styles as there are yoga teachers, so find a teacher that you like. I really like yin yoga, where you hold positions for a longer period to stretch out muscles and your fascia. You often work with props to support your body. Some postures can be a bit painful in the beginning, but when you feel the release, it is lovely. Slow hatha yoga or yoga flow can be a great option, or if you like more powerful movements and posture, you can go with that.

The great thing about yoga is that you work the positions with your breath. You start a flow in your body while working with your breathing, which helps loosen up tightness and blockages. Many women have tried yoga, but if you haven't, give it a try! There are many studios that offer prenatal classes as well.

CRANIOSACRAL

Craniosacral Therapy (CST) is a gentle, hands-on approach that releases tensions deep in the body from pain and dysfunction and improves whole-body health and performance. It was pioneered and developed by Osteopathic Physician John E. You lay down on a massage table with clothes on, and the therapist works on you by holding on or above your body. Sometimes, you can feel or sense a stronger reaction. Sometimes, you don't feel much at all. I have been nauseous, dizzy, relaxed, tired, and felt happy or not feeling anything during these sessions. It is different from time to time, but it supports your whole-body health and calms down your systems if you are stressed.

VITAMINS

Vitamins can be something to consider. If you are trying to get pregnant, it is recommended to add folic acid, and your doctor will know this. Folic acid is important in red blood cell formation and for healthy cell growth and function. The nutrient is crucial during early pregnancy to reduce the risk of birth defects in the brain and spine. Folate is found mainly in dark green leafy vegetables, beans, peas, and nuts.

Multivitamins are a way to get extra support from all the vitamins and minerals that you need. Even if you eat healthy, varied foods, you can benefit from some extra support from a multivitamin, especially during wintertime. There are a lot of vitamins and minerals to support your body. If you choose one, make sure it is a great brand. It is like a jungle. You must follow your own gut and feel what is important to you. Vitamins and minerals cost a lot of money, so be mindful of what you choose and why.

While you are trying to get pregnant, folic acid should be added. Folic acid supports the cells and makes red blood cells. It also supports the development of the fetus. The recommendation is to start a couple of months before your pregnancy so your levels are good to avoid spinal cord injury of the fetus.

Here is a list of the most important vitamins, minerals, and corresponding foods that provide you with them:

A - Pumpkin, egg, tomatoes, spinach, broccoli, beef, carrots, pepper

B2 - Quinoa, eggs, lentils, avocado, spinach, wild salmon, almonds

B3 - Lentils, turkey, portobello mushroom, sunflower seed, beef

B6 - Green beans, banana, carrots, avocado, eggs, chickpeas, spinach

B9 - Lentils, egg, lemon, broccoli, asperges, red beet, Brussels sprouts

B12 - Egg, wild salmon, liver, sardines, dairy, sardines

C - Pineapple, strawberries, broccoli, kiwi, lemon, pepper, parsley

D - Egg, sardines, wild salmon, fish liver oil

E - Almonds, sunflower seed, hazelnuts, avocado, kiwi

Calcium - Sesame seeds, cheese, lentils, almonds, figs, spinach, chia seed

Magnesium - Fish, nuts, and veggies

Zinc - Fish, nuts and veggies

As you see, if you eat a variety of food, you get a lot of vitamins. Keep in mind that today, for many reasons, food does not contain as many vitamins as it used to, especially during wintertime. Much of this issue is due to the poor quality of our soils. It is a good idea to add a supplement. Maybe you need other vitamins or minerals, too, but I just wanted to show you where to find the most important vitamins for a balanced body.

WATER

I will again emphasize the critical importance of filtered, healthy, quality water as a critical way to best support your body. Drink a lot of good, filtered water. With help from the combination of water, exercise, enough sleep, and deep breathing, you help your body detox and recharge. Your blood fluid volume levels increase substantially when you are pregnant, so preparing for this by drinking a lot of water all day long only helps to feel your best and be your healthiest.

HERBS

There are many herbs that can support you and your body. For example, a cup of herbal tea can calm you down if you are upset or have a headache. A cup of chamomile tea helps you relax and is great before you go to bed. Dandelion is great for supporting the liver and kidneys. Dandelion supports the lymphatic system and helps with periods. You can eat the leaves in a salad or dry the whole plant and use it in tea. I buy dandelion online and use it as tea or coffee, warm or cold, depending on the weather. Oregano supports your body to fight bacteria and viruses. Adding fresh or dry oregano to food is great. If you would like to add natural herbs to your diet, that would be a great way to support your health and healing. Research more about different herbs and how they support you. There is a lot to learn.

FOOD AS MEDICINE

Food, what you eat, and how you eat are critical to health. How you fuel your body is critically important. You can do a lot by investing time in buying organic or local veggies, meat, eggs, and other products. It may take a bit longer when you grocery shop before you know where to go and where to find your stuff, but it is so worth it. It costs a bit more money, but you must consider what is important to you. The organic food is often a bit more expensive but also without all the extra poison you don't want in your body and system. Locally grown is also a great option.

The next thing is the time you also need to invest time in preparing your food and cooking from scratch. If you are used to buying prepared food, you just heat up or order home from the restaurant. It will be a bigger change, but you hopefully find joy, calm, and excitement to prepare your own food. One great aspect to preparing your own food is that you know exactly what it is made of with no extra unhealthy ingredients that are considered gross. There are many tips and tricks as to how to manage your week with preparing your own food without spending hours in the kitchen. I know you want to do other things too. In my life, one of my great joys is having friends over for dinner, when they arrive, we enjoy some snacks, and a glass of wine, and I hand over a cutting board and knife, and we help each other out preparing dinner and having a great time together at the same time! Also, there are a lot of recipes online and a ton of cookbooks. If you would like a kick start to this process, I have put together a two-week meal plan with a grocery list. Easy, tasty recipes with leftovers to make your daily life easy and smooth. You find a link at the end of this book!

Life is too boring without treats, but if they are kind of healthy, just enjoy! Great food made from scratch supports your body if you want to get pregnant and live a great life! It is most important to have a variety of food, so having treats every once in a while is ok. Food that does not spike your blood sugar too much and keep you full and energized for several hours is also most beneficial. It is good to mix different meat with a lot of veggies, fruit, berries, and nuts. As always, you have to find your way and decide what works best for you. If you are willing to invest time in preparing your food, it will pay you back with better health, better energy levels, more glow in your skin, and a happier you!

During heavy, painful periods, it helps if your zinc and magnesium levels are good. You find zinc and magnesium in fish, nuts, and veggies. Great fat from salmon, nuts, and olive oil helps your hormones, and vitamin E from seeds and avocado can reduce pain and bleeding. In other words, it is critically important to be aware of and in control of what you eat to support your body, hormones, and period. If you are interested in learning more about how you can support your body with food as medicine, there is a lot of information to look for, and one option is to start with my little two-week quick start.

ALCOHOL

During pregnancy, I chose not to drink any alcohol. It wasn't a difficult decision for me, as the health of an impending pregnancy, as well as hopeful babies, took precedence. I must admit that I really enjoy a glass of red wine when the weekend comes or a glass of champagne as my go-to on a Friday! But, when I tried to get pregnant, I reduced my intake of alcohol in the beginning of the trying stages. I did not cut it out because my philosophy is that you need to have some joy and treat your soul right. A glass of something you really enjoy now and then does not hurt. French women drink alcohol during pregnancy, as far as I know. But I didn't want to risk getting my body and eventually, a baby getting any kind of harm just because I wanted a drink.

THERAPIST/COUNSELOR/LIFE COACH

When I went through IVF, there was an abundance of feelings and thoughts. Being emotional also happened quite a bit. I got a therapist to talk with to help me and support me. I think this is a really good idea. You can benefit from someone to talk to, from outside of your family and closest friends, who do not judge or know you at all. But it must be öhe right person. You must feel that it is a match and that you can release your heart, worries, and concerns with that person. I did not get the right support from my first therapist and stopped. Years later, I got the opportunity to talk to a physiatrist in Germany, and they had a different approach. I was given a lot of names and numbers for references, and I could check their home page and location. I went to three different therapists and found a lady that I liked. I ended up seeing her for two years, and she helped me a lot and gave me a lot of tools to handle trauma and different topics. She also had different meditations and breathing exercises to help calm down my nervous system.

REIKI HEALING

The word reiki means mysterious atmosphere or miraculous sign. It is derived from a Japanese word where "Re" means universal and "Ki" means life energy. Energies can be stagnant in your body and block your meridians. A reiki professional will help you with this, which results in healing your pains and moving your energy to where it is meant to be. Reiki is a way to help your body heal. The healer works on balancing your body and loosens up blockages. Your energies will be more balanced. You really benefit from going deeper and working with your inner child and trauma. It can be hard work to face your fear and your inner demons, but it helps you understand what triggers you, why you act as you do in different situations, and what you have taken with you from your childhood that you are not aware of. This is a great way to start new patterns and heal the inside to be able to move on without blockages and some trauma.

ENERGY MEDICINE

Everything is energy. Working with someone who can support you to get the energy moving and your blockages loosened up and disappear will give you a new life experience. It is incredible how much you can do on your own to support your body and mind. Start each day with a small exercise to get your energy, balance, and calmness going at the same time. It is easily done by tapping acupressure points that connect with the meridians and lymphatic system. At the end of the book, you will find out how to do an energy hook up and balance, as well as calm and Energetic your body. I share with you some points you can hold to support your pain, cramps, and heavy bleeding during your period.

It could be a great idea to get an energy medicine treatment. Donna Eden is a woman that healed herself via energy medicine, from a difficult disease that the doctors had no way to cure. She uses her life to live and teach the power of energy medicine. Many other people also speak and teach about the power of energy.

PILATES

Pilates is an exercise that helps you strengthen your core. With a stronger core, you have a straighter posture and less pain in the neck, shoulders, back, etc. It also helps tune your body and get stronger and more flexible. In Pilates, there is a saying; "Less is more." I like that. It is the small adjustments, sometimes the small movements, that make a big difference. With a straighter posture, you automatically get better self-confidence. I started with Pilates after one of my surgeries, which was recommended by a doctor. I got hooked and had so much fun, but it was also hard work. I went on to earn my Pilates Instructor Certification. It has helped me in many ways, and I suggest you try it to see if it is something that speaks to you. I don't like gym and big group sessions, so this was something for me. I love the small Pilates and Mindfulness classes that I teach. I have taught in Sweden, Germany, and the US. Also, you can find a lot of it online and on YouTube, so check it out. I share the same classes on my home page if you are curious about my sessions!

BREATH WORK

Breathwork is also a big tool. Our breathing is important. Most people do not breathe properly. We are stressed and only breathe short breaths in the upper part of our bodies. There are many ways to breathe to help our bodies release stress, tension, and pain. It is also a great tool for relaxing our bodies and getting more oxygen so we feel better, and it helps our bodies heal.

One easy tool I use is the quick-fix Breathing Minute. For one minute, you close your eyes and take deep breaths through your nose and out your mouth. You breathe in and feel how your lungs, diaphragm, and belly fill up with air. Hold your breath shortly, and then slowly release the air all the way out. Put one hand on your chest and one on your belly to feel how it expands in and out when you breathe. You only breathe 3-4 breaths for one minute, maybe less. Try to do the Breathing Minute for a week at least 2-3 times a day and notice how it affects your body and mind. We must be better and good at using the small, easy tools that help us feel much better. If your system is calmer, you have better focus, are more relaxed, can handle situations better, and will have better sleep.

LYMPHATIC DRAIN MASSAGE

Our lymphatic system is important for our health. The lymphatic system transports all the slog from our organs and cells out of our system. If the lymphatic fluid is slow moving, it takes longer to clean our bodies. It can easily build up stagnation or blockage and cause pain and illness. Maybe you have had or have some tenderness around your armpits or around your neck. We have bigger nodes there that easily can get a build-up of fluid and feel tender. In our bodies, everything is connected, and if we have a healthy lymphatic flow, all our organs are happy, including our reproductive organs. You can book a lymphatic drain massage to support your lymphatic system, but you can also do a lot at home by yourself. At the end of this book, I explain some movements you can do by yourself to support your lymphatic system.

CHINESE MOXA

I went to a workshop in Sweden to learn about Chinese medicine and how they use Moxa. In China, they use this a lot, especially to prevent diseases. It works on the meridian system, and you feel better and look healthier when you do it on a regular basis. One session takes about one hour. You do it in the comfort of your own home. It is preferable to do it outside, but with cold weather, you have to be inside. It smells a lot, and my family is not so fond of it. You make a little ball and then put it in a seashell that lays in sea salt in a little hat. You light the ball on fire. I always light mine outside. When the ball is black, you put it on your stomach below the belly button. It can get quite hot. I have a T-shirt under the hat. The heat starts movement in the meridians, and the ball burns out after about one hour. Then you throw the aches away outside. It warms up your whole body and starts processes. For example, it loosens up blockages that make it easier to transport slug out.

SAUNA & INFRARED SAUNA

A sauna is one way to boost your immune system by helping your body to start producing more white blood cells. When you enjoy a sauna, your muscles soften and relax, and your body detoxes. You get rid of old skin cells and feel and look healthier. Infrared saunas do the same but also work on a deeper level and help your muscles recover.

MUSIC & CRYSTAL SINGING BOWLS

I guess you have noticed when a song you like starts playing on the radio, your energy changes, and you feel happy. Music has a big impact on our mood and body. The frequency the music sends out responds to our bodies and cells. Some people can get emotional from a symphony orchestra performance. They play at 437 MHz, which is a great frequency for our bodies. Crystal singing bowls have the same frequency, 437 MHz, and can start healing and wellbeing in our bodies. Maybe you would like to try going to a symphony concert or a singing bowl session. They have other frequencies, too, such as 437 MHz. You can feel the same happiness and wellbeing at any concert. Music touches our hearts and souls. Just as we can turn on sad music to help us release sad feelings, we can turn on lovely music to help us feel good. When you feel low next time, turn on some music you know you like, even if you don't feel like it. Turn the music on and give it a try. Your energy starts shifting, and you feel a bit better. If you are really low and sad, try to turn on music and dance and let all emotions out. Nobody sees you, so why not try? It can be a fast way to release the feelings you have and change to feel better!

Chapter 8
Partner Relationship and Pillar Support

"Stop finding ways you can't do something. Then you're not going to do it. Find the way that you can and then go for it."

— Isa Rae

This chapter will help you to mindfully think about and plan your support network, referred to as your pillar support. Think of a large, heavy building being constructed. It has to have pillar foundational support to survive, last, endure, and be of use. This applies to your journey as well. Having a dedicated, caring group of people to help you and your partner through the ups and downs of your journey will be critical to helping you maintain a healthy mental and physical state. Most people do not give this aspect of their lives much thought or attention. For stressful experiences, taking the time to consciously think about this aspect of your life will provide you with many benefits.

Having heavy and painful periods and/or endometriosis is difficult enough to manage, let alone manage it by yourself. It is so important to inform, talk, and share what you are experiencing with your partner, hopefully, some close family members, as well as some close friends. Choose your closest friends with much care. Make sure you know you can count on them no matter what. It is far better to have a few friends or just even one best friend than a lot of people who don't understand, can relate, or support you properly. This one friend or the few that you choose wisely become(s) your "inner circle" of pillar support.

It is also helpful to know that there are close confidants you can call when you need to talk or can join you if you need to go to a doctor's appointment or the hospital. Make a list of these people. Some will be in your inner circle, and some will be on the periphery of that circle. Nonetheless, thinking about this ahead of time and making a list is important. It becomes part of your "tool kit" to help you manage the ebb and flow of this journey.

There will be days that you don't even feel like handling daily tasks, like going to the grocery store. Your pillar support folks can bring some food or a treat to cheer you up. As you go through the days, weeks, and months, some of the peripheral folks – like maybe a neighbor you don't know that well – may become part of your inner circle as time passes and trust builds.

SELF-SUPPORT

There are ways that you can support yourself too. You can have meals prepped in the freezer (and some ice cream or chocolate or what you like for a special treat). You know that some days can be harder than others, so make special arrangements for yourself to feel as good as possible on those days. Maybe call a friend over to help you clean, or to do laundry together so you can visit and pass the time. Talk to your partner a lot about what you experience and be sure to tell them how they can make it better for you. Do not assume that they know. They are going about their lives in parallel with yours and they will not always be able to be fully in tune with your vibe. Be sure to show your partner much appreciation either when they are supporting you or right after. Either way, it is important that they know that their efforts are being appreciated.

ASSISTED REPRODUCTIVE TECHNOLOGIES (ART)

When you enter into the phases of assisted reproductive technologies or treatments (commonly referred to as ART), your support group becomes even more critical. Day-to-day and needle needed, going through ART and surgeries with unhealthy reproductive organs involved is really like treating a disease. Most people do not realize this, but think about it for a moment. Your body/my body was not able to function in a healthy and normal way. Therefore, medical treatments had to be applied to help my body along to perform like it was created to. Having a supportive environment is worth gold, and even better is having special people in your life that show up as your angels.

Sometimes you get support from unexpected ways or persons. I had a colleague that I had worked with, but only for a short period, and when I was on sick leave a lot due to heavy bleeding and IVF treatment, this wonderful woman stepped up and showed me unconditional love when I had a hard time. There was one occasion when I had to go to the hospital for urgent surgery. I knew she did not like hospitals at all, and yet she chaperoned me with care and love. Not only did she stay by my side the whole time, but she also pampered me in her apartment for a whole weekend following my hospital stay. I did not expect that love or caring support, but it was amazing, and it still touches my heart deeply. Some people are angels on earth. Open up to be supported from unexpected ways and unexpected angels.

Here is a prayer to support you when you need it:

I need to always remind myself that the Divine (Higher Power, God, Spirit, Source, or whatever you believe in) is with me, walking beside me and making a way of escape for me by lining up people, places, and situations to bring me out of my tough places and into a place of strength. I do not have to allow fear to paralyze me. I am not alone.

— A prayer shared by a wise, loving mother

CLUBS, ORGANIZATIONS, & ASSOCIATIONS

Be sure to check out where you can join endometriosis clubs and buddy up with others who are going through the same thing as you. These associations are in most countries. You can become virtual buddies with someone whom you can also receive a lot of support from who is also going through IVF, as an example. As a member of these types of organizations, you have access to information with Awareness Months that are celebrated. Endometriosis month is March. One year, I gave a supporting membership as a gift to some family members who were part of my pillar support team. These types of funds go toward research. Different countries offer different associations, and in the U.S., there may also be state-level groups.

Do you already have any friends that you can talk to openly? Does your partner have friends to talk to? What about family members, immediate or other? In my case, we did not have any friends in our new country, and we felt lonely and nobody could understand. This is why I stress this part of your planning so much. I wish I would have taken the actions to set in place a support network.

TOXICITY

The other aspect to mindfully picking your pillar people and support network is to remember that some people can be hurtful. Do not allow this toxicity in your space in any way, shape, or form. Examples include the hurtful sentiments that were shared with me in the past by my "friends." Comments like: "Your period can't be that bad." "Come on! Let's go out dancing. It will do you good." Or "It can't be that hard to do an IVF treatment. Soon you will walk with a stroller." Or, the best one when you are swollen and feel like shit; "Oh, are you finally expecting?" I got the last one several times and I will never ask a woman if she is pregnant even if it is obvious. She must tell me.

Just as it is critical for you to form your pillar support network, it is critical for you to seriously level up your communications with your partner. For example, when you and your partner are about to start an IVF journey, there is a lot to go through and talk about to ensure you both are aligned with your understanding.

What do you want to do? Are you both for an IVF?

It is important to **express your feelings** and what you want so you both know what you are okay with doing and what not to do.

- **I wrote a love letter to myself!** I hid it in my drawer, and a year later, I opened this letter. It was so lovely to read the kind words I wrote to myself about what I wanted to achieve, what I was ready to invest in this process with all my mind, body, and soul, and to remind me of what a good person I was. I suggest that you write yourself a similar letter. Outline what your goals are, why, how, and when the hormones are raging and you reach a breaking point, retrieve this letter, and read it. This does not have to be a one-time occurrence either. Tuck the letter back away for the next time it is needed. Maybe add to the letter as well!! This letter is a reminder, during the process, to yourself as to why you embarked upon this journey at the beginning. We can forget when shit hits the fan!

- Do you have the **time** you need to invest (scheduling and going to doctor's appointment, blood draws, scheduling and taking your meds)? You may both need help and support with all these kinds of things, as the process affects both of you, your schedules/work. Your partner, as example, will have tests to take as well.

- Are you both okay with knowing that there will be many rough days and some better days? You may need time to recover from the rough ones. It's good to be aware of this and that it can turn into a lot of recovery time. Does your work allow this? What is your **price tag for becoming pregnant**? How much are you able/willing to invest?

- The two of you (partner relationship) need to come to terms with the fact that over the next month that you are involved with an IVF process, your **lives as you know them really do not belong to you anymore**. You need to let go, fully offer your whole selves up to this process because it all belongs to the hopeful baby to be. This may seem harsh, but a lot of your life (social, work, friends, family, etc..) are superseded by the demands of the IVF process and the demands on both of your bodies.

- **IVF costs** a lot of money. You need to discuss how much you are willing to invest. What about alternative methods like adoption or surrogacy? Are you both willing to spend money on this? Why or why not? Hopefully you reach your goals, but there is not just a one-way street. The common thing is that they all cost money.

- What about your **insurance** in the country in which you reside? What will they cover? What will they not cover?
- Also, give some consideration to any **alternative** treatments you may want to have to support your body while you are going through procedures.

Add these costs into your calculations. They will help to optimize your body. You need time and money for that as well.

- Be sure to **prioritize your partner relationship**. How can you support each other the best during this time? Write a list with what you like the most/ appreciate from your partner and what they can do for you. Simple things can help a lot like a little note on the table when you wake up and your partner has left for work. Or it makes you really happy when your partner brings you a small gift, or even just cleaning up the kitchen, bringing you a cup of coffee/tea. It is often that we appreciate different things. Some prefer a do-er and some more emotions and affirmations, etc. It is great to see what your partner likes the most and try to do that for them. Normally we treat them with what we like for ourselves.

I put small notes and treats in my husband's bag and all over.

He is more of a doer and did a lot of cleaning and organizing. I appreciated it, but he knew it was also really special when he left a note on my nightstand when he left early. Knowing what our partner really enjoys makes it easier to do that for them now and then. It is the small things in life that means the most. Taking good care of each other and support and carry/lift the other one when its down and other way around. To give and share energy with each other. Support each other's ebb and flow. Accept and respect of feelings at different times.

It can be hard to not feel guilt or shame. It can be challenging to not blame your partner. Decisions and choices will have to be constantly made and finding fault with each other does not help at all. When something is discovered about the other person (physical limitation) you may become resentful, and this reaction may well indeed be surprising to you. How can you, for example, feel resentful if there is also something medically wrong with your partner?

Going through an IVF treatment also has a psychosocial strain that affects your intimate life. It can be hard to be intimate and enjoy sex when it has so much focus on reproduction and whether or not the sex will result in pregnancy. Nothing is fun if you must do it on a schedule with pressure. To not be able to have kids of your own and to go through IVF is comparable to serious diseases and other life changing diseases. It can be helpful to have a therapist to talk with. Your health and the person you know you are will change a lot with the hormones, and you don't recognize yourself anymore and must find a new orientation how to accept yourself and your body. Many women describe how they don't recognize themselves or their behavior after starting with the nose spray.

You do not have control over your own body and feelings. Feelings you don't know where they come from pops up. It can be hard for your partner and people to understand. It is hard for yourself to understand what's happening. Your life is in someone else's hands. You feel robbed in many ways. I remember feeling that I will never have a loving, passionate night the miracle happened. I won't be able to think back on how I created something with love and passion. Instead, I ate, breathed, and lived IVF. IVF becomes your identity. It is a lot for the woman but also for her partner.

It should be standard to inform couples at an IVF clinic how much an IVF process affects their relationship, feelings, social life, economy and at what times it would be good to stop. As a couple, you both need to agree on what is your limit, like we will do three tries then we need to focus on us, our relationship.

OTHER OPTIONS

There are other ways to be a caring, loving human during this time of life. Adoption, surrogate, foster, extra aunt, get a pet, are some examples. It hurts deeply when reproduction does not work, and you feel left out. What should be normal is not happening for you and you can feel jealous, anger and many other feelings. It is not easy for partner, family, and friends to understand and support the best way. The more you communicate the better results there will be. There will be people that do not understand, and I suggest do your best to keep distance or not talk about the subject when you meet.

Keep your relationship with partner and closest friends and sisterhoods close and be open to support and some criticism that is meant to be supportive. By keeping it real, open, and honest, you will feel the best. I also want to share that I truly think an IVF baby is so much more loved, if that is even a possibility with a new born! The parents put in extreme efforts to make it happen. It is wonderful with each and every child, but an IVF child is a love supported miracle.

If you have any religion or spirituality, this is a good time to use it. Whatever you believe in or rituals you have they can support well during this time so keep going. Your best friend is yourself; I encourage you to turn inward and listen to your heart. It can be tricky to hear your inner voice at start and to know what you want. But if you take a moment to slow down and listen to your own voice that will be the best way for you. All people you ask for advice tell you what they think is the best and it is great to get input, but you have to decide for you.

I have been able to create a list of my advice regarding support. Here it is:

- Listen to your own heart.
- Communicate with partner and friends.
- Make a list of what you need/want when life is hard.
- Choose your support friends wisely.
- Consider a therapist/ life coach.
- Get an online, virtual buddy system.
- Stay off line and limit googling after you've completed your initial research. Instead, talk to your medical team or support women who have gone through the same experiences. Google can become a negative rabbit hole quickly.
- Join an association that can support you.
- See if you can find supporting sisterhood IRL (in real life!) or online.
- Put a note on your mirror with something supportive. Maybe "Good morning, beautiful," or "You are awesome" "I am worthy and I deserve to feel great in my own body." If you read a pampering message every day, you start a new pattern that will boost your self-confidence. Who does not need that?

Chapter 9
Beyond Fertilization

"It actually doesn't take much to be considered a difficult woman. That's why there are so many of us."

— Jane Goodall

Wow! Can you believe you made it this far? Congratulations! What a journey you have been on too. Believe me, I know. This has not been an easy feat in any way, shape, or form. There are so many days, weeks, months, and probably years where you have been working toward being at this point in your life. How ironic, too, when you reflect back on your earlier life, where you were probably doing the opposite like I was: trying to prevent pregnancy! Remember the days when you were possibly hassling with birth control pills, the removal of your diaphragms, or spending money on condoms? So much of our time, mental energy, and resources went to *avoiding getting pregnant*, and now you are on the flip side.

This chapter, Beyond Fertilization, is about the four stages you could possibly experience in your journey after IVF. Here they are:

#1 Fertilization was not successful, and there will not be any embryo(s) transfers(s).

#2 Fertilization was successful, and one or more embryos were implanted in your uterus.

#3. Maybe you had a successful transfer and were pregnant but had a miscarriage like I did. Or,

#4. You are successfully pregnant.

Wherever you are, please do not, for one minute, think this is the end of the journey or lose hope. There are so many remaining possibilities and roads you can choose to take from wherever you are at this point. I would like to talk about miscarriages though. I'd like to share my experience of miscarriage after IVF. **You can completely skip this part if you'd like**, but some info is being shared here in case you are in need of it.

MISCARRIAGE

First and foremost, miscarriages after IVF are common. Please know that I am not saying this to take away from the emotional toll and mental struggles we experience after a miscarriage. But it's important to know that it is common. Regardless of all the medical assistance and high-tech procedures, keeping the embryo "viable" after conception isn't as easy as some people think. I had a miscarriage after my first successful embryo transfer and implant and that makes it harder to stay positive and believe that a new pregnancy will still happen.

Let me share with you some more details around my one and only miscarriage experience. After the first successful harvest, when I was around thirty-four years old, one embryo was success-fully implanted in my uterus. When it was time for the official pregnancy test, four weeks after the transfer of the embryo, it showed positive! We got happy and felt relieved as well! A few weeks later, around week six or seven, I started bleedings again. I couldn't believe it! I felt so sad but was reassured that this can happen and not affect my pregnancy. With this news, I did not give up hope. It remains interesting to me that I was able to keep hope, renew hope as well as sustain some kind of hope within me after all I endured. I believe this to be a saving grace for me because I was always a person that chose to believe in the good in this world over the negative.

The bleedings continued, so I called my doctor who instructed us to get to the hospital. It was there, at the hospital, where they could not see any signs of life in my uterus by the ultrasound procedure. I was told "there is nothing there." At this time, the embryo should be between an orange seed or a blueberry attached to my uterus, along with all the nutrients and blood because organ development had begun.

I was given a pill to promote the continuation of the bleeding to "clean me out." They told us that it was a miscarriage. I hadn't really even begun to fully believe that I was pregnant, when all of a sudden it was taken away from us. My sadness continued to grow. Just the imagining in my mind that there **was** a life that had started but was stripped away. It all was mind-blowing. I kept thinking that we just were so happy when we got the two blue lines on the pregnancy test that indicated pregnancy. It was a lot of feelings tumbling around in my body and mind after the devastating news. Sadness, anger, fear, feeling left out, *WHY? WHY ME? WHY US? What did we do wrong?* People that don't want kids, end up having some. Addicted people have unexpected pregnancy, and other couples get pregnant seemingly "just by looking at each other." But for us, who had been longing to start a family for so long, it was hard, painful, and even shameful. I told myself not to feel ashamed, but with my body not working like it "should," it just hurt so deeply inside, it became easy to crawl behind a wall of shame.

We had a little life that just started, but for some reason, it could not stay with us. I think it was some meaning with the miscarriage but at that time it is hard to take. If it is a miscarriage, it is nature's way to solve when something is not right. (or just teach you a lesson!) My body was sore from all the hormones, and I felt so sad and angry as well because it seemed like I had done all this treatment for nothing. You are sad because you just lost a baby and then we top that off with continued heavy bleedings that make you feel even worse. I also remember thinking at this time that I actually now hate pregnancy tests! Why should I like them? They only make me happy or sad, and the happiness is so short lived because it doesn't last. They also cost money and I didn't want to spend one more cent on a pregnancy test. What a peculiar, recurring, obsessive thought I had rolling around in my brain during a crisis situation! I put all my anger on the pregnancy test kits! And what did they do? Probably laughed at me with no positive results and by saying: You wasted some more money by buying me! I continued to have these thoughts and even found myself laughing at them. But, unbeknownst to me at that time, I actually would never ever buy another pregnancy test in my life. How ironic life can be.

TRY AGAIN

We left the hospital with the news that we could "try again" whenever we wanted. You just start at it again. For most couples, they are instructed to wait a bit to rest and to accommodate other medical recommendations. But for us, we went straight for it! Because of my bleeding, my body was not able to rest and so we were told to just try again. When your body is not able to recover, as mine was not able to, there is no reason to wait. We followed the doctor's recommendation to just go for it, without any hesitation or pause. We got the only frozen embryo that survived out of five, that survived the thawing process. It was transferred to my uterus, but this failed miserably. It was at this time that I just wanted to fully give up. But my husband insisted that we give harvesting one more try and that we do not give up, that we continue moving forward with our dream.

From a health care perspective, the government was paying for most of the services I have been describing. We, however, did have to pay out of pocket for much of the hormone treatments. We realized how blessed were to be in a country where such services are provided. This last harvest was covered by the government, so from a financial perspective, we had nothing to lose and possibly a baby to gain.

And there it was, our Hallelujah moment!! We were blessed to become pregnant from our last embryo transfer that was the result of our last harvest This was after I endured all the steps in the IVF process once again, with embryo transfer process endured three times. Three times for both the IVF series as well as three embryo transfers! Isn't that insane? Sometimes I felt insane!

The series of these procedures are emotionally and physically uncomfortable. The steps you take build upon each other as you go from one step to the other. First come all the hormones, as discussed in the IVF chapter. I had to take drugs over a three-week period, each of the three tries. They suppress your normal ovarian function while the series of injectables stimulate my ovaries. My husband had to endure the sperm gathering process multiple times as well. The sperm needs to be "washed." The semen is separated from the sperm and chemicals are also removed as they could be harmful to the uterus. This sperm washing part of the process helps to enhance the fertilization capacity of the sperm.

Egg retrieval had to be repeated three times as well. They aspirated eggs from my artificially stimulated ovaries by using an ultrasound guided needle vaginally. Needless to say, I was extremely tired both in body and mind and was losing hope, but it was my partner/husband who didn't give up! He lovingly convinced me to go through the IFV process one more time for a one last try of an embryo transfer. We were fortunate enough to have this last try financially covered by the Swedish government as the last of our three. I was a bit concerned and kind of scared because now I was going to have to go through the entire process once again. If we had any left "in the freezer" to use, doing this again would have been avoided.

With our partner relationship being as close as it was, my husband knew me well enough to know that if we didn't use our last, government provided chance, I would have regretted it later. This was a true test of our closeness, our love, our support for each other as well as deep trust. It was also a testament to our ability to keep the lines of communication open and to ensure we communicated all the time (as covered in my Relationship and Pillar support chapter).

When we did the last IVF, we had already endured the long process of signing up and being approved for adoption. Let me tell you, there was so much paperwork and the process itself is rigorous. But this was our Plan B. In retrospect, I truly believe that having this adoption process ostarted was one reason why this last try was successful: I had relaxed a bit because we already were into our backup plan. The deep stressors that I had been dealing with non- stop for so many years were calmed down by me just knowing that there was another plan in fruition for us to be gifted a baby.

Maybe you have back up plans as well. They could include adoption, like we had agreed to be our back up plan. We also had researched going the surrogate route, but I was not convinced that I physically and emotionally endure another egg harvest. We lived in Sweden, and you had to harvest the eggs in the country where the selected surrogate lives. But there was an even bigger problem. Surrogacy was/is not legal in Sweden, so this made the option of surrogacy not viable for us. There were other different options and other solutions in that particular country, like using my husband's sperm and a donated egg. The upside to this way is if we went this route, I would be spared from doing another egg harvest. But after I reflected on this for a while, I truly realized that I wanted a baby through my own experience of pregnancy. I think many people would like to have a baby of their own if it is possible. That was my first, most natural choice.

After several years of heavy bleeding, different hormones, and the entire IVF process, I had a stressed out with a worn-down body. How I was capable of maintaining somewhat of a normal life during these years of trial and error remains a mystery. But somehow, the last IVF try was successful! We got pregnant! At first, we were both so elated. The dedication we maintained to making our dream come true seemed to pay off. However, we soon realized that my pregnancy was not unfolding in the ways we had expected. This was upsetting. I finally got pregnant and was waiting for the glow to appear and the wonderful state so many women experiences. But again, for me, it was filled with too many ups and downs.

I did not feel sick in the mornings, nor did I throw up like many women do the three first months. Instead, I was plagued, once again, with heavy bleedings. This drove me crazy because I thought every time I bled, we had lost the baby. This happened several times and each time, I felt like I was having another miscarriage. I spent some weeks in the hospital on three different occasions during this second pregnancy. I was in much pain, did start to suffer from nausea and almost fainted several times. On the mental and emotional level, it was hard to believe that the pregnancy would go full-term. It was hard to feel excitement and joy because I was scared all the time, surviving one day at the time. I hope you are not experiencing this as well, but if you are, I hope you find comfort in knowing that I went through this.

Many years later, I read my diary from that time of my life. I didn't understand at all how I managed to endure and to do all that was required of me. The constant adjustments, pain and surprisingly, the loneliness I felt that no one could understand how lonely, scared and sometimes sad I was. Of course, I was happy that I was pregnant, but I was not sure at all that it would end well. On the outside, as usual, I showed a happy, strong face. In my head, I would tell myself that after all this time with bleedings and IVF, it was fantastic that we were pregnant. But me, the real person experiencing it all, was downright beyond exhaustion and dreamed of a long break from it all. I never said this out loud to anyone before, nor did I share it with even my husband. Don't get me wrong, I was so grateful for this pregnancy, but the price my mind and body had paid was too high.

YEARS HAVE PASSED

Many years have passed since this time and I still am working on recovering. No one told me how hard the hormone treatments impact your body and how long you need to heal from them. And then we have the emotional and mental traumas. There is a lot to heal from. With the different stages or modes that our nervous system can be in, I realize now that I was in a long state of what is called freeze mode. This can also be referred to detach mode or shutdown response, in relationship to a person's nervous system status. I noticed myself shutting down, checking out, or disconnecting entirely from the rest of the world. I felt numb or empty at times, along with my mind feeling blank. I struggled to connect with my thoughts or feelings or verbalize them to others, while feeling strains of apathy, depression and demotivated. Seriously, this was not at all what I expected to be feeling when I finally got pregnant. Then again, when I took a few minutes to reflect, I realized that for the last five years of my life, I was not only trying to get pregnant, but I was also in survivor mode. It makes full sense now to me.

Regarding one's body when being in the nervous system freeze mode, you can generally feel detached, apathetic and may even feel depressed and/or unmotivated. My muscles were generally weak and felt fatigued and heavy. I felt physically exhausted, energetically depleted, or mostly numb and unable to feel anymore emotions. I was more on the silent side, and when I did have to talk, my speech was monotone and forced. I remember feeling unsure of what really were the next steps in our process and how real my pregnancy really was. I remember also having difficulty concentrating on tasks or thinking clearly and critically.

After a normal pregnancy and childbirth, it's not unlikely that many women have some kind of experience on the trauma spectrum, be it small or large. But, when IVF is involved, the chances of experiencing heavy trauma on another whole level increases. Many women go through IVF much easier and smoother than me I have noticed, but I think there are many women having a lot to work with after a bleeding and/or IVF journey. I believe that my journey was on the much more challenging and sad side, yet I realize that many other women have similar experiences. It is common to feel that you have no control over your own body. The hormones make you act and feel so many feelings. You react with irritation, anger, or tear up constantly to everyday things. If you would like, you can read excerpts from my diary at the end of the book, as I did write down what happened. In my diary, I talk about the group I joined online that was expecting the same time as me. With them, I could share some feelings, ask questions and we gave ideas and shared information with each other. I suggest joining a group like this for support, especially if you are on bed rest or can't go out that much. It is important to have someone to talk to and share experiences with that are in a similar situation, in addition to your pillar support and inner circle.

I do specifically remember feeling worried when we decided to do a blood draw to see if there were any indications of Down syndrome. At that same time, they also measured the baby's neck and did an extra blood draw to collect data on many more medical condition indicators. But the big question is what **you** as parents decide to do with the information. I suggest you talk before the test and agree on what you both think, feel and what you would like to do when you receive the results. We also chose to do an organ test. Even here you need to talk about what you feel if something concerning shows up.

We did not check the amniotic fluid because of the risk of miscarriage. We wanted to do checkups to see if the baby is healthy but did not gamble with losing the baby via amniotic fluid draw risks. And to be honest, I was not about to have that long needle in my abdomen. To this day, I still do not like needles at all. You may think you get used to them, but not me. I accept this about myself and I honor it. I also realize that this is a trauma wound that I still need to work through. I have taken many blood draws since IVF, but I don't like it.

When I developed thyroid trouble after pregnancy, I had to have a lot of blood draws to keep an eye on the levels. After several years with synthetic and natural thyroid hormones, I worked with an alternative doctor for some years, and I do not take any medication for my thyroid anymore. I want you to know that you can heal from a lot of issues. Your body wants to be in a state of equanimity. As of today, seventeen years after my pregnancy, my last physical checkup blood draw resulted in all levels being normal. Vitamin D and Zink were a bit low. Considering it was the fall season, it was good to know this to level those up for the winter. It is a good idea to get your annual checkups, but I know and feel my body and follow my intuition much more now a days and it is often quite spot on!

After IVF, most countries keep an extra eye on the pregnant patient to see that all goes as it is supposed. We were blessed to be pregnant and with twins! It was a lot to take in but wonderful news. Excitement mixed with fear and worry. I ended up with bleedings three times during my pregnancy and that add to the frequent checkups. I think it is quite common that becoming moms, with endometriosis, have some issues during the pregnancy, but this is not always the case. Most women with a history of endometriosis have a normal pregnancy and can enjoy the process. Women that have experienced miscarriages have trouble with not obsessing and worrying during a pregnancy. Be gentle with yourself where ever you are. Remember to have self-compassion and grant yourself a lot of grace every single day. It's only human to have such worries.

Every country has different approaches when it comes to giving birth and the delivery room. It is good to research what the options are, specifically for where you live. What kind of painkillers do they use? What kind of different approaches during labor? I gave birth in Germany and thought that it would be the same as in Sweden, especially since the countries are neighbors. But boy how wrong I was! The things I had planned for did not exist in Germany and it was too late to change to return to Sweden, so I had to change my expectations.

For my delivery, I wanted the birth to be as natural as possible and my husband and I were communicative around this topic. I was open to sharing what my expectations were and my husband assured me he would do all he could to make that happen if I could not speak for myself. We also practiced a lot of breathing. In the beginning, I could not do the breath work for long at all before I got dizzy, but it got better. In the delivery room, I was planning on doing the breathing to support the contractions for a whole minute with only 2-3 minutes in between.

PREECLAMPSIA

Unfortunately, I got preeclampsia. Easily explained, my body attacked itself and the only thing that helps is to get the baby out. Preeclampsia is when the placenta starts to not work properly and cannot support the baby with nutrition and oxygen. It is not known why preeclampsia occurs, but particles from the placenta and baby leaks into the blood system and starts an inflammation. The doctor measures blood pressure during pregnancy, and if it is consistently too high, preeclampsia could be starting. Also, if there is protein in the urine, the indication of preeclampsia becomes stronger. Your doctor should be checking your blood pressure as well as taking a urine sample at every checkup.

Preeclampsia can develop slowly, but also fast and can become serious within hours. Twenty years ago, many more woman and babies died because of preeclampsia. Today the doctor can see indicators in blood pressure and urine early on. Still today though, many women and babies pass away every year due to preeclampsia. I have also read that preeclampsia is associated with higher risks of stroke or heart, vascular diseases later in in the woman's life.

Hemolysis Elevated Liver Enzymes Low Platelet Syndrome (HELLP) is considered a more severe form of preeclampsia and unfortunately, I also developed this syndrome. It consists of Epigastric (abdominal) or substernal (chest) pain, including abdominal or chest tenderness along with upper right-side pain from liver distension. The red blood cells break down. Red blood cells need to support the body with oxygen. Nausea, vomiting, or indigestion with pain after eating is common symptoms. Many get bad headache that won't go away, even after taking medication such as acetaminophen. Edema (swelling) is also common.

As these symptoms continued to take over my body, I felt more swollen from water weight gain the last days prior to labor and it was harder to move and bend my knees walking the stairs. The morning that I had an appointment scheduled with my German ob-gyn, I thought it would be good to take a bath. I remember looking so odd and so funny in the tub! We had a quite deep tub, but my belly was so big, had to use a wet towel on top of it so I did not get too cold! I was pregnant with twins and quite big but not a giant. Little did I know that this bath would be the last one I would enjoy for a long time.

At the ob-gyn, I got called to the office at once without doing the normal routines. They had taken a blood draw to check my liver levels because I had told them that I was getting itchy, which can be a sign for severe preeclampsia. The doctor came in, shared the results with me and promptly told me to go straight to the hospital delivery room. My initial response and outburst were "But I haven't had lunch!" How funny is that? The ob-gyn told me I could have something to eat, but then to go straight to the hospital. On my way to a restaurant, I called my husband who was four hours away and in a work meeting. I told him I was on my way to the hospital and that he had to come as soon as his meeting was done.

I remember going to a yummy sushi restaurant because I had read that miso soup is good energy and had a mama sushi plate. A Mama sushi plate is with avocado and not raw fish that pregnant woman is advice to prevent. I was a bit tired and even if it was a short walk to the hospital, I called a cab. A new friend called who had heard about my situation and told me not to go home and grab my bag as I had planned. Instead, I should go straight to the hospital and she would meet me at the entrance. What a gift that was. After arriving at the hospital, we got a room immediately but there was so much paperwork to sign that I did not understand it at all. Maybe this, too, is something to prepare for ahead of time. Go to where you will delivery and talk through all the paperwork. Maybe you can receive copies ahead of time and have them all filled out prior to even going! How relieving would that be?!

We spent four full hours in that room. I had monitors on my abdomen so we could follow the heartbeat all the time. I was blessed that my friend helped out, including calling my husband because there was no Wi-Fi in the delivery room. Long after the delivery, my husband told me that she had asked when he would be there because I had started to change color and she did not want to be the only one there when I delivered. She was afraid that my husband might not make it in time for when the babies arrived. She knew that with preeclampsia you can get a little changed skin-color and that it might be an urgent c-section. She herself had experienced preeclampsia and an emergency c-section. She wanted to make sure that my husband would soon be arriving. Finally, my husband came, and I had got medication to slow down the process.

LABOR

If the babies stayed one more day, we would be in week thirty-seven and the lungs would have been fully developed. It is best if babies do not arrive before their lungs are fully developed. I got a room and had to stay overnight, and my husband was sent home. I had so much abdomen pain and especially up on my ribs. I later learned that is a sign of preeclampsia and HELLP syndrome. I walked the hallways up and down and finally could get some sleep for a few hours with a heating pad. My husband came in the morning and then we went back to the delivery room. Unbeknownst to me, when we arrived, the medical team asked me why I had not told them that I was having contractions every five minutes. I had not told them because I did not know! I had anticipated and expected that my contractions would come and go. Instead, for me, there was just constant pain. I felt stupid! No one had told me that it was possible to just have constant, devasting labor pains that don't stop all the time.

We were able to go out for a short walk. The weather was nice and warm for the first day of November. The sun came through some clouds. We walked in the park with many colorful leaves on the ground and saw people walking, talking, or biking to their jobs, enjoying their lives. I heard birds twirping and kids laughing in the distance. I was hanging onto my husband when the contractions came. I thought now we are close to delivery. My water still needed to break and I remember thinking that it would soon be over. We returned to our assigned room. Then the doctor enters the room and clearly announces: "The babies need to come out NOW." I did not get any explanation, just that it was urgent and they wanted me to sit in a wheelchair to go to my room for preparations for the surgery.

I wanted to walk but had to make stops at every contraction. It took too long, so they got a rolling bed and took me back to my room where a nurse shaved me down there, put on a hospital gown and then the rolled me to the surgery room that was prepared for me. I later learned that the babies were under too much stress and did not get enough oxygen so their heartrate went down. My blood pressure had started to rise. My husband was shown to a room to get changed to surgery clothing and told to wait there until someone called him. He later told me that he felt lonely and that he wanted to be with me to make sure I was ok. I can only imagine how he felt so helpless, just waiting, and not knowing what was going on.

They helped lift me over to a surgery bed and then I had to try to sit up and curl my back like a cat. That is easy with a big belly!! I was scared. What I did not want was a c-section and a long needle in my back and here I was about to experience both! The anesthetic doctor was professional. He was tanned with blond hair and looked like a cool surfer. He talked in a way that made me feel a bit better. He talked a lot and he was good at making me think of other things with his questions. They washed my back with a brow/yellow fluid. It is to disinfect. They told me to sit absolutely still. I had a nurse in front of me and she told me I could hold on hard to her hands. Gosh, I squeezed hard as they gave me a numbing shot and even harder when they had to use the long needle for the epidural. I never saw the needle because I was looking at the smiling nurse and closed my eyes for a while. I still admire that nurse that just kept smiling and did not say anything about my hard squeezing. It must have been painful. Then it was over and they told me to lay down. I started to be numb at once and could hardly move my legs back up on the bed so the nurses lifted them and then they quickly rolled me into the surgery room.

There was a lot of people in the surgical room. I could not count them all. It was weird because they were all strangers, in a room with me, where the most intimate of experiences was about to happen. They put a big green curtain in front of my face to almost block my vision, but mostly to keep the area sterile. They put one of my arms out on each side like a cross. My midwife nurse aunt had told me before that during a c-section, you sometimes can see what they are doing because there is this large, silverish lamp that reflects like a mirror so you can see a little bit of what's going on. But unfortunately, I could not see anything except the green fabric.

MEATBALLS

I will never forget one of the medical team members! Thank God for some comic relief from him during this time! The anesthesia doctor had realized that I came from Sweden and told me that he used to go to IKEA and enjoy their meatballs. He was wondering if he pronounced meatballs right in Swedish! He did not, so I taught him. You see, he was great at distraction! My husband finally arrived. Thank God! He entered the room with his quick, familiar steps with a nurse that told him to sit on a little stool next to my head, on the same side of the green curtain that I was at. Our eyes met and funny as it is, the first thing out of my mouth was to tell him how I had just taught the anesthesia doctor how to pronounce meatballs correctly in Swedish!" Isn't this all so bizarre? As if that wasn't enough, I actually had the doctor demonstrate his "meatball" Swedish word skill to my husband!

I then asked my husband if they had started the section and at the same time, we heard a splash. Wow they are moving fast! One nurse came with a baby wrapped in a towel and touched the baby's chin with mine. Then she and another nurse run away with both babies. I got a tear in my eye and at the same time felt tumbled like a rock in a stormy ocean. I could not move my arms and dry my chin off from the baby's wet cheek. A nurse told my husband to follow her. We had a beautiful boy and a girl! They told us that they seemed to be alright. I can't recall that any of them were screaming or made any noise. It felt like a short time but it took about one hour to finish the c-section and I was taken to an intensive station in a single room. From the stress and the preeclampsia, I had some black outs and can't remember it all. My husband filled me in a lot later with all the details. He was taken to the delivery room that we have had and the nurses let him help when they checked the babies" length and weight. They told him that the babies where big for being twins born one month too early. Then they left the room so he could say hi to his children. He felt overwhelmed and confused as this was not the way it should be! We were supposed to be together to greet the children. Here he was standing alone with two tiny babies and did not know what to do. He had put the camera in his pocket so he remembered to take a picture. I am glad he did that because that is the first photo of our babies when they are about thirty minutes old. When I first saw them, they were already over an hour old. To this day, I do not know which baby I got on my cheek in the surgery room. Was it my precious girl or my precious boy?

My babies were taken good care of that night, as far as I know. I can't remember why, but neither me nor my husband were with our babies that first night. I had many concerns about that later when I thought about it, but the babies had good care and were with each other while I was recovering. My husband was sent home. That night was the longest in my life that consisted of so much pain, freezing, sweating like a pig, a headache from hell, dry mouth, and as soon as I almost fell asleep, the blood pressure measure equipment would beep and wake me up. I was on many medications, and the antibiotics were working to heal my infection.

I had hoses and things attached all over my body. They had a big can on the floor I realized in the early morning, and it was full of urine. I lost a lot of water that night from sweating and urine through the catheter. I wanted my husband and kids to be there. Why was I here alone? I needed them. This is not how it should be! I had thoughts crossing my mind that I needed to survive this. Nobody told me how bad I was and looking back, I am glad they didn't. I think that would not have helped. My liver was fighting for survival. My whole body and all organs where fighting. HELLP syndrome is a rare but life-threatening condition in pregnancy. It causes red cells in the blood to break down. It also causes problems with the liver, bleeding, and blood pressure. I lost a lot of blood as well. All together this made it life-threatening.

INTENSIVE CARE

I ended up at intensive care. I really was hoping for a normal birth after all we been through. In Germany they have a fridge to store champagne or wine in the hallway of the delivery rooms. After giving birth, it takes some time for the milk to start being produced so the Germans celebrate with a good drink if they like. I think it's cool that the hospital has a fridge for that reason. They also say that it supports the process to start produce milk! My husband collected my champagne from the fridge some days later, and it was still there!

We met at the intensive room. The German nurse asked me if I wanted to breast feed and I said yes. The babies were laid down on my chest. In Sweden, Germany, and the United States, you have almost the same gown with buttons in the front or back depending on how you put it on. That is the thing that is common for the countries. It was interesting to see how the babies moved to the breasts. It was week thirty-seven, four weeks too early but the first day that the lungs were developed so they did not need any incubator. They found their way and got some drops.

This is where my husband and I experienced the most frustration with the language barrier and challenges. The medical staff should have told me that if I had planned to breastfeed, it would be best to try to focus on my recovery as well to be able to take care of the babies. But they did not tell us in a way we could understand! They did not speak any English and I thought I understood German quite well, but not all the terms they used in a hospital were German words we were familiar with. My husband did not understand the German language there either. We did not understand well and could not catch up what the staff was saying to each other. It would have been better if we had understood the language better. The staff was not good with English either. That would have been helpful.

My two beautiful babies were taken to the children's station and my husband was sent home. This is when the horrendous chills began. I started to freeze. My teeth were chattering, and I had to concentrate to keep my tongue in the middle of my mouth and not bite myself. I had equipment attached to my body all over like in those hospital series on TV. Every thirty minutes, my blood pressure was taken automatically and it started to beep. My blood pressure was way too high. I was the only one in the room and I could see a control room and they had all my stats and care under their control. After the freezing slowed down, I started to be super warm and began sweating so profusely, that the sweat was running down my whole body. The nurse took my temperature and it was lower than normal, resting around 95F. This seemed so strange to me because I was physically sweating. Shouldn't my temperature be high? Since I worked in the ski patrol, I knew that your body can react in this manner when under stress, infection, or injury when you are out in the cold weather. This was not good because when you sweat that much and at the same time the body temperature goes down, this indicates that your body is starting to shut down. It is like that when you freeze to death. You start to feel warm and to undress.

As you are reading this story, isn't it just quite unbelievable how one thing after another kept happening? Just like before my pregnancy, one thing after another would happen before, during and after labor. I was numb with disbelief while this all was going on. Soon enough, I started getting horrible pain again. But this time, the nurse told me to tell them as soon as I felt more pain. When I did, they came with a big syringe and I thought no, not another one, please God! But they took one of the four hoses out from my hand and put a different fluid hose in with some sedation and pain killer. I could feel the cold fluid go up my arm. Then it felt better. With the high blood pressure my body could not take more pain than it would rise.

I almost passed away that night. It's a surreal thing to even be saying, let alone knowing. That was the worst night in my life. It was supposed to be my happiest, but I was fighting for my life, fading in and out of consciousness. I got little rest, was obsessively thirsty but was not allowed to drink because of chances to throw up. I asked if my sweet, precious babies should come to breast feed, but was told that they were fine. Some weeks later, I was told that it was not safe for me to have my small babies in my arms as my arms could cramp up and injure or even kill my kids. So, the babies had to stay away. Thank God they didn't share that with me at the time. Newborn babies are fragile and I could have squeezed them to death.

I was fighting terrible headaches the first couple of days and could not tolerate any light. We had to keep the room dark. But the fever and chills broke and I was on my way to recovery versus survival mode. Day three or four was the first time I saw my babies naked when my husband changed their diapers. It was terrible the first time I had to go to the toilet. I think it was day four or five. A nurse came and helped get my legs to the side to help me sit up. With one nurse under each arm, they checked that I could stand on my legs and then I could lay down again (totally exhausted) and she took the catheter out. I asked her what to do when I need to go to the bathroom and she told me it was time to try that when I needed. Gosh, that was quite an adventure taking a few steps to the toilet by holding onto the wall and slowly sitting down with much pain. My roommate told me to keep the supporting band around my waist even if it was a bit stiff, but it helped.

I stayed at the hospital for ten days. Every morning, I got shots in my upper legs to keep the blood thin so I would not get a blood clot while laying down. The shots stung like an angry bee sting for like an hour or more and left me with big bruises. Two weeks after, when my mother was able to visit, she was shocked when she saw how much my legs were bruised and looked just horrible. There were so many different bruise colors: purple, blue, yellow, red, orange, black and so on.

GOING HOME

They checked the liver every day. The first day I was allowed to go home, I went home. I met my midwife in the corridor and she had an outburst asking me, "what are you doing?" I told her that I was going home, and she asked me to consider staying a bit longer, but I wanted to go home. I had been sharing a room with three different ladies, and I could not sleep well. My babies needed to be breastfed every second hour. I wanted peace and quiet.

With endometriosis, it is common to have thick, noticeable scar tissues. I did get a thick scar from the c-section. I didn't practice much yoga before I got pregnant. I started after giving birth when I was allowed to do the after-pregnancy exercise. It felt good to do soft movements to help the body getting back on track.

I noticed when we were supposed to lay on our stomach on the floor that I could not do that. It was painful. The teacher told me that we had to let the c-section scar take its time to heal, so I got a pillow to put under me so I could lay down without discomfort. It was also tricky to do some of the movements. It felt like I had a rubber band in my tummy. Every time I tried to reach tall, it pulled me back. I had my husband adjust the height of the changing table several times for the babies since my back hurt that much. I thought it was my back that had to have the right position, but it was actually the scar tissues from my c-section that was pulling. It was when my midwife came home and treated me with a reiki healing, we started to understand the problem. She told me that the energy was just going up to my waist and then circled back to my feet. It is supposed to flow from feet to head and back. She looked at my c-section and told me that her husband, an ob-gyn, had to have a look at it. After that treatment, I got fever and felt sick again for three days. I understood that this is a serious problem.

When I met the new ob-gyn, after he examined me, he said that this scarring was not good nor healthy for me. The scar tissue was thick, raised and red. The name for this condition is hypertrophic, where your body creates much more scar tissue that what is actually needed. This type of scarring can cause inflammation that is dangerous to any future pregnancies, cause adhesive small bowel obstruction (ASBO), chronic abdominal pain and create difficulties for any future surgeries that need to be performed in that area. So, here we go again, planning for yet another medical procedure.

During this precious time of healing, recovery, and new parent time for me, both sets of parents were working fulltime in Sweden, which made it challenging for any of them to provide a lot of support. My husband was working long days and traveled quite a lot leaving me alone with the kids for most of the time. I found some college students and a "rental grandma" that could support me a little bit here and there.

After one year of this way of life, where it felt like I was sailing my own ship through a web of currents that constantly over powered me, I felt done. I became depressed. I did not enjoy life even with two lovely babies. They were beautiful, but they never slept so neither did I. An easy way to break down a person is through sleep deprivation. I became anxious ridden and was afraid of myself, that I might mess up and hurt the kids. I did not dare go out on the balcony the first year because I was afraid that I might slip and throw the kids from the balcony on fourth floor. Many women think these things and actually feel like they are going insane. I now know that I wasn't experiencing post-partum depression. Instead, I was in what is called "birth psychosis," an actual mental illness that affects a woman in the first weeks after birth.

BIRTH PSYCHOSIS

With birth psychosis, symptoms appear suddenly and you lose your sense of reality with mood swings, delusions, etc... Being sleep deprived, breast feeding two babies, trying to recover all by myself when my husband went back to work, was just way too much for me. Nobody understood how exhausted and depressed we can be. I did not tell my husband in the beginning because I felt ashamed. My nervous system was completely de-regulated. But when I told him, he could not really understand the serious-ness in what I was telling him.

The first year for me, post-delivery, was foggy. I don't remember much. I was there. I did all that you are supposed to. I had strict routines to help me survive. Family and friends were wondering why I had to be so strict and change both diapers at the same time, breastfeed both at the same time, eat at the same time and go to bed at the same time. It was because I was in full survival mood. I fell in my bed as soon as I put the kids to bed and somehow cleaned the kitchen and prepared their bottles for the early morning.

I still had the critical scar tissue to deal with form my c-section. Before the surgery he told me that I could probably leave the hospital after one day. I ended up being there for a week again. I remember that it was a beautiful day in the beginning of June when I walked to the hospital at six o clock in the morning. The sun was shining, and I felt safe with the doctor and was looking forward to less backpain in the future.

We started to plan for a surgery to remove scar tissue. I got the surgery when my babies became toddlers at the age of one and a half years old. My IVF ob-gyn, whom I went to before pregnancy, referred me to a clinic. I remembered to tell my IVF doctor about my back problem, and he told me that it comes from the scar tissue. So, prior to the surgery, he told me that we could soften the tissue. At the clinic, we tried to reduce the hardness in the scar tissues by injecting cortisone. He pinched me with the needle and injected fluid about twenty times along the scar tissue. The scar tissue was as thick as my index finger. It was painful. I had to focus on breathing, and I was cold sweating during the process. I was thinking, **why** am I doing this? I questioned if it would help me.

I can't recall how many times I went there for this treatment, but it was several times and each time painful. I remember the doctor injecting me that he felt my pain as well. I could see it in his eyes. The progress we thought could be made with this softening approach wasn't coming to fruition and I ended up having to have the surgery anyway. I had it all cut out, which meant that II had to go through all that cortisone shot pain for nothing!

Interestingly enough, I learned from my ob-gyn that did the surgery that the scar tissue line was low on my belly, actually down in my bush. This was because both of my babies" heads were low in my abdomen from as early as half way through my pregnancy, so they had to cut the c-section low. I woke up with a drain next to me. Fluid needed to come out from the wound. It took a long time for it to heal. The doctor told me that this surgery was worse than the actual c-section.

During that following summer, there was a small piece of the wound in the middle that took a longer time to heal. A lot of yellow fluid was released several times and once again, I found myself lining my underwear with pads, which brought back horrible memories for me. The Band-Aids were tricky and painful to remove and replace as well for my wound care. One time, I put the pad on a scale and the fluid weighed more than twenty grams. But I am a survivor, and this too did pass. Today I have a scar that is deep into the skin. The doctor had to carve out a lot and all the attached fat cells too, so my lower abdomen looks a bit weird. But this is nothing people can see even when I wear a swimsuit. Some swimsuits cover the scar better than other because of its deep line. I also still suffer from some nerve damage in the inside of my right thigh from the c-section cuts in my lower abdomen. This is actually quite common, I have learned.

I was hoping that the bleedings would be better after pregnancy because that was what I was told. That was not in my cards. When the babies were about six months old, my doctor told me that it would be best to start back on birth control pills or if I didn't, the bleedings would continue and I would also most likely have a hormonal spiral. I choose the hormone spiral possibility because the mere thought öst going back on the pill was beyond my comprehension. I was, after all, supposed to be past all of that.

I got my period back shortly after I stopped breast feeding, when they were six months old. Quite fast, the bleedings got heavy and painful. I got cysts and had to see the doctor often again. When I came to the office, they had often burst, and he could only see fluid in the pelvic area. A friend of mine read about endometriosis and sent me the article. I put a check on all symptoms. I found out that there was an endometriosis (endo)clinic close to where we lived. One out of two in Germany. I called and got a first appointment. My husband went with me and when I told the doctor about my symptoms, he stopped me after a short time and said that this indicates endometriosis, and we need to do schedule a laparoscopy. I told him that I had asked my ob-gyn if he thought it could be endo and that he had said no. He could not see that on the ultrasound. This doctor laughed a bit when I told that and told me that many are not aware of endo and its symptoms. Normally you had to wait for six months to a year for your laparoscopy, but they wanted me back in two weeks. With two small children and this heavy bleeding, many cysts, pain, and headache that gave me a heavy, tight iron helmet (it felt like that) was too much.

We paid for extra insurance so I would be treated by the professor doctor who did the most surgeries. I came to the hospital in the late afternoon and slept there since I was the first patient in the morning. The surgery started early, and when I woke up, and a nurse asked me how I was, I could only say that I wanted to see my husband and had a lot of pain. My husband entered the room, took my hand, and stroked my head, and I got something injected in the needle in my hand. It felt good, and I slept again. I didn't want to be alone like I was after giving birth. The next time I woke up, the nurse asked if I was okay with moving to my room, and I asked the nurse to get my husband to comfort me. This really helped me. I asked if I could get the same painkiller there then I would like to move. She told me that that was not possible. I understand addicted people better now. That stuff (I guess morphine) took away all the pain.

They rolled my bed into the room, and I stayed there for five days. Again, with a drainage hanging on my side. It was much pain. The evening before I held my hands on my abdomen and said goodbye to my uterus, if it had to be removed. The doctor had told me that if the uterus was bad, they could remove it at the same time instead of during a new surgery. Some women do not feel like a woman after removing the uterus. For me, I think I got my life back for the second time after my uterus was removed. I could not take care of my kids with this heavy bleeding and pains when I had my uterus. I was also depressed and did not want to live.

It is common that you get depressed with endometriosis. Without a uterus, your hormones spiral out of control. I began a dark time with a sad mind. I was convinced that the kids would have a great life without me. I went to psychotherapy for some years. Birth psychosis is a level-up from birth depression. Birth psychos can appear after giving birth if the person has hormone issues and little sleep. The person can get anxiety, worry, depression, despair, and suicidal impulses. I am glad I had that high threshold in my body that I did not do anything harmful. I never wanted to hurt my babies, but I did not care about myself. I don't wish anybody to be down in the dark, black hole. It takes a long time to crawl back up. It is especially challenging when you wish to never return.

Looking back, within ten years, I had endured five critical abdomen surgeries as well as having to remove a big cyst that got attached to the ovary, stomach wall, and bowels after my hysterectomy. I have a lot of scar tissue in my body today, and sometimes, with bowel movements, I get pain. Sometimes, it is like something sharp is stabbing me, and I need to hold on to something and breathe. I am now fifty-one years old and feel ok. I still work on releasing some trauma to feel my best.

During the first year after the uterus removal, I was so very sore and sensitive down there. In combination with less sleep, and a slowly developing depression, we did not have any intimate times or sex life. In looking back, I know that both my husband and I were longing for being loved and to be held. With two small babies, my healing, and my husband's full-time demanding job, we had our hands full. There was little time for any partner time and it was not easy to get time to take care of your relationship. Adding to this was the fact that we did not have any relatives close by. I should have asked for more help.

We aren't always great at asking for help. Women are used to managing most everything on our own and trying to live up to being invincible. Where we lived, they had a program with "rental grandma." We applied and got a grandma: A retired person who was looking for grandkids and families long for a grandparent. Both are matched together. That was awesome that someone could take the kids for a walk for a couple of hours now and then, giving me some much-needed quiet time and restful naps. It is a great idea, and I hope it spreads to more places.

Going a little further out into "Beyond Fertilization," I want to share that due to all the stress my body endured for decades, I developed several autoimmune diseases, along with thyroid challenges and gluten intolerance. It is all related to a stressed-out body. When our bodies are stressed for too long, our adrenal glands get fully burned out, and our organs get worn out. They can compensate for a while, chugging along, but then they deteriorate in some way or another, one after another and we get more and more sick. Now, in present time, if I don't fully rest and take care of myself, I get body aches, easily come down with a cold or get downright sick. Two years after pregnancy and one year after giving birth, I had eight sinus infections in one year. It takes time to build up your body after too much stress, but it is possible. I have focused the last years on balancing activities, building my body back up, and resting.

By sharing my journey after the IVF and Beyond Fertilization chapters, I hope to open the eyes to people that endometriosis does not end with the use of birth control pills, pregnancy or with a partial/full hysterectomy. I wish the world would start taking women's health much more seriously. We need more information, research, and a lot of more understanding and caring. I also advocate for much more support and help with utilizing alternative treatments while fully embracing a healthy lifestyle. We need to open up to new ways of healing. Pills and surgeries are not the only answer.

Chapter 10
Conclusion

"You define your own life. Don't let other people write your script."

— Oprah Winfrey

I have re-experienced so much by writing this book in both good and bad ways. I am proud of myself for writing this book and am so glad I did because the book-writing process that I endured allowed me to heal a lot more deeply throughout its various phases. Writing this book, paragraph by paragraph, chapter by chapter, word by word, made me realize just how much I have gone through. Frankly, I am surprised I survived it all, literally and figuratively. Looking back, I realize that I almost didn't when I almost died after giving birth.

I have gained a much deeper understanding of endometriosis, IVF, treatments, surgeries, healing, spirituality, energy, chronic health issues, prematurity, medical team challenges, depression, issues with lack of sleep, and much more. But I have also learned how strong I am. I am a **Warrior Queen**, one that never gives up, no matter what. A ***Warrior Queen*** who got to experience her pregnancy and its joys while embracing the small wins along the way. I got to feel, gratefulness for shared hearts pumping in my abdomen, deep emotional healing with my partner, and experience the powers our bodies have.

One aspect of myself that went unexplored for most of my life is the natural whims I have toward playfulness, singing, dancing, and much more like painting. I have been painting now and then for many years. I hope you like my painting on the front cover of this book. Creating art is a way to work through my feelings and find that bliss state where time just fades away. I often think that what I paint is not good, but this ego response only teaches me the importance of not comparing myself with others and, instead, being kind and gentle with myself. Many friends and people have told me they enjoy my paintings and that is wonderful. Most important is that I enjoy painting and it supports my life journey and gives me joy. This is why I selected the painting I did for my front cover: Mirakel. It represents my miracles, by babies when they were still inside me and I had so many emotions. I felt excited, scared, happy, and grateful while I was painting it.

I did not have knowledge, understanding, or information about endometriosis while I was growing up or even into my early adulthood. I did not know anything about this disease. Still, to this day, I have heard that it can be inherited, but we don't know. No one in my family has had endometriosis. In earlier generations, this was not something you talked about. As you know by now, after reading my book, one goal I have is to keep up with the research, knowledge, and understanding of what continues to be discovered. I have a teenage daughter, that I want to

have the best support if needed, and there are way too many women suffering. My deepest wish is that women read this book and gain a lot of new knowledge, help, and support.

It is devastating that more emphasis in the science, technology, and research arenas are not focusing more on endometriosis and other pelvic, women-related health issues. It needs to happen much faster. Endometriosis is more common than diabetes, and the percentage of women having difficulty getting pregnant keeps rising. Writing this book will help bring these issues to the forefront and support my fellow sisters. This was of utmost importance to me as well.

Going through what I did, or any parts or pieces of it, is difficult. It is difficult to see your way to a better life when you are in the middle of so much pain. But please know, especially after reading my work, that there are tools, people, and other resources to help support you. Your journey through your days and your life can be bearable, one step at a time.

For me, looking back, I can honestly say we felt almost thrown into IVF. Everything went so fast. I was stuck with bleeding, a weak body, and just wanted a solution to put an end to it all. By reading this book, I hope you know much more now than you did when you picked it up. I hope you also know where there are still knowledge gaps that need to be filled with more information before and during your journey.

At the hospital, when the twins just were born, a nurse told me that they are scorpions, and they are and would be strong children. I liked that and still remember that moment. I innately knew that they were strong because they started fighting for survival right when they became into being, in my belly. I am grateful for all that my kids have taught me.

Both my kids and I were often sick the first years after they were born. Then, their first year in childcare was when they turned three years old. The longest stretch that they managed to be in day care was for three weeks in a row during the whole first year due to ear infections all the time. When they started school, we soon learned that something was not as it should be. There was something not quite "normal" with both of them. We saw many doctors and experts and undertook many holistic treatments. Soon enough, both kids were diagnosed with dyslexia and one with ADHD and the other ADD.

It is not unusual that IVF kids have a higher risk of being born premature and sometimes with some type of health issue. Many that I know, including my own, have ADHD and/or ADD, attributes that I prefer to call "superpowers." These superpowers vary and are unique to each IVF child. I would love to see more research on the similarities and differences between kids from IVF and regular pregnancy. Maybe it is just what I have come across in my life, but I guess some more people would like to know. There is an excellent review article from The National Library of Medicine, National Center for Biotechnology Center from 2020, entitled ***Long-term Health of Children Conceived after Assisted Reproductive Technology (ART).*** It concludes that there are no associations between ART and ADHD or ASD for singleton babies, whereas for ART in general there is an increased risk. Here is a snipped of this article:

The aim of this narrative review is to summarize the present knowledge on the long-term outcomes of children born after assisted reproductive technologies (ART). The main outcomes covered are neurodevelopment including cerebral palsy, cognitive development, attention deficit hyperactivity disorder and autism spectrum disease, growth, cardiovascular function, diabetes type 1, asthma, malignancies, and reproductive health. Results have mainly been obtained from systematic reviews/meta-analyses and large registry studies. It has been shown that children born after ART, when restricted to singletons, have a similar outcome for many health conditions as their spontaneously conceived peers. For some outcomes, particularly cardiovascular function and diabetes, studies show some higher risk for ART singletons or subgroups of ART singletons. The fast introduction of new ART techniques emphasizes the importance of continuous surveillance of children born after ART.

Here is the link to the full article with all its glorious details. With more knowledge, you have more power and will be more empowered. Take a read and dive in!

https://www.ncbi.nlm.nih.gov/pmc/articles/PMC7721037/

When our children were little, while we were driving, it was common that we had conversations with them that extended for long periods of time! On one side, they told us that they both were sitting on separate clouds, and it was on these clouds that they both chose us as their parents at the same time. We had not talked with them about religion or spirituality, but I could clearly envision this scene in my imagination and loved it! Their little voices told my husband and me the story as easily as if they were describing the color of their shoes!

The younger generations listen more to their bodies and their needs. I am grateful for this. I want my kids to live a life they enjoy, with gratitude and boundaries. Our kids taught us to listen to ourselves, slow down, enjoy the moment, and much more.

Since this is the conclusion of my book, I would be remiss if I didn't share with you the things that I would have done differently if I had the chance to go back in time and do it all over again. After a lot of reflection, here are the magic ingredients that I would work hard to incorporate into my journey:

- **Research** - Do a lot of research before, during, and after all phases of the journey.
- **Endometriosis Info** - During my time with heavy, debilitating periods, no one mentioned the word "endometriosis" (and that was over several decades). If I had any awareness at all about it, I would have spent so much time researching it, talking

to others who had it, and seeking specific expert help. KNOWLEDGE IS POWER!

- **Listen** – It is so important to deeply listen to your body and heart. Everything works better when we are aligned with our hearts. I just did what the doctors told me, even if it did not feel good sometimes physically and/or emotionally. In hindsight, I can say that it actually felt like I was being violent to my body. But when you are desperate, without knowledge, you do anything to be free from what is bothering you.

- **Courage** – In retrospect, I wish someone would have talked to me about courage. I wish I had more courage to listen to my body and heart and try to find other ways and solutions that could work better for my body.

- **Alternative Treatments** - I would have tried alternative treatments, like Reiki, energy medicine, and other holistic treatments to heal from the inside out first.

- **Food as Medicine** (not medicine as food) - I would use food as medicine. Maybe tried to find a professional health coach to support and help my body heal with the right foods. Food has a critical impact on our bodies.

- **Self-Care & Self-love** – I would have taken better care of my body, mind, spirit, and heart while being intentionally gentle and kind to myself. Doing it over again, back in time, I would sprinkle daily doses of grace into my routines as I made mistakes, faltered, and fell down. I would clearly respect all that I tried and would be more grateful for everything that worked out. More of an effort would have been made to celebrate what's working. Doing more to pamper myself to increase my self-esteem is on the list as well.

- **Lighthearted** - Try not to take everything so seriously - It is easy to be serious and focused on what to do, what the next step is, and constantly finding new solutions, so much so that you forget to enjoy life and have fun. The hard stuff is there no matter what we do, so we must remind ourselves to have fun and not to take so much so seriously. our bodies heal with music, dance, laughter with friends, and other things we enjoy. More of the fun helps you heal!

Find your unique recipe that works for you to let go and relax more in the joys of life. We each are like our own unique soufflé, one of the most difficult of desserts to master. Even if you do everything right, and it rises in the oven, when you take it out, it can still collapse. Then you start to ruminate and think and think, what is it that I did wrong? It's best to just move straight into trying it again. Discover new tricks along the way so you find your special recipe that works for you.

During my journey, I have tried my best and experienced a lot. With my twins being sixteen years old now, I am now enjoying and experiencing a much different life full of gratitude. To understand my kids better, I figured out that I had to start to work on myself, my own healing of trauma, to be able to support others. It is ongoing, and I am still eager to learn new things about myself, life, healing, health, and all that makes life interesting and fun.

We can heal much in our bodies. For instance, I know today that the painful side of endometriosis subsides with much better, healthy nutrition, movement, breathing, and reduced stress. Even if I don't have bleeding anymore, endometriosis never disappears from my body. It is a chronic, life-long illness. It is important to continue to support my body the best way I can.

Also, this topic is so critically important, and I wish I had been aware of it a long time ago: your gut health. We need to understand how healthy or unhealthy our guts are. If we discover that we have leaky gut or other gut issues and we start healing our gut, that seriously helps so many other parts of our bodies to function healthier, like our liver and lymphatic systems. It can also lead the way for the hormones to work better. Everything is connected and will work well if we give the right conditions. I wish I had known more much earlier in life. I'm grateful that I can share my knowledge now and pave the way for someone else.

It was exciting to experience so much during my journey writing this book! I learned by experience how much thoughts and feelings are connected to our bodies. When writing, I got severe period pains, the same pain I had long ago when I had cysts that burst. It lasted the same as before, about three days. I could not believe this was happening and I thought this is for real and scheduled an appointment with ob-gyn. Everything was fine and my thyroid and hormone levels where fine. I learned that we could experience severe pain and trauma when we open up that feeling or thought. This was yet another lesson I learned. It is good to know about how our bodies remember and keep the score, somehow "fooling" us! But we can also heal it and leave it behind.

CARRYING A HEAVY HEART

Now and then, memories from the past still come up to the surface. My depth of sorrow is still in me. It bubbles up, and it comes in waves, almost like how grief works. These different feelings remain capsulated in my body, just like they will with you. This is also a lesson learned.

Shared Heartbeats

When I was in the middle of it all, the warrior within me kept strong. This is common for many crisis situations, stressful times, or traumatic experiences that last a long time. We remain strong as warriors during those times, in "survivor" mode and protection mode, to get ourselves through them. Now, I have the time and head space to work on healing the sorrow, the frustration, the anger, and the irritation. These feelings got stuck in my body, and there were small blockages in different body parts. I needed to release them. I survived all these years, but the energies from these deep emotions are still in my system. The trauma, the change, all that I went through scarred me and does not just go away. The young me, the woman in my twenties and thirties and the woman I am today, all these versions of myself are impacted I am all these women that it took to be the woman I am today. Now that I am not in survival mode, now that I have the knowledge and the strength to heal, what was encapsulated in my body can be released! Now it is about joy and moving forward.

I am blown away by how much magic we are surrounded with. I successfully treat my daughter's heavy bleeding and horrible pains that last for a week at a time. I get scared that she will suffer from endometriosis the way I have. I treat her with energy healing, and in about half a year, we went down from seven days to about five, and to almost no pain or pain she can handle. What a blessing. She doesn't miss school anymore due to her periods, either. We are breaking the cycle already! She was skeptical toward my healing at first, but one day, she was in so much pain that she let me treat her the first time, saying, "-Do whatever you like, Mom." It worked. By the next period, she came to me and said," Mom, can you please do your magic again?" Even if you are not a believer of this, you can heal and get surprised at how much it does for you and become a believer.

I live a soulful life as a soulful entrepreneur. All the experiences I went through over so much of my life and so much of my adult life, the creativity, risk, imagination, courage, hope, and faith, led me to where I am today. Here I am, concluding the conclusion of my first book.

Life is beautiful. I encourage you to enjoy this journey we humans call life, to the fullest. Don't care about small triggers. They are not worth it. Reach out for all the support you need and can afford. Be true to yourself and live your life. Be the best YOU! Choose how you like to start your day, every day. You can arrange your mind to make each day count.

I believe in you.

You can believe in you.

Be the warrior you are for the girl you left behind, the many versions of yourself you have been since, and for the woman you are now. Take her hand and walk together to find what you need to heal and thrive, inside out. Keep love as your guiding light, for yourself, for others, and for *Shared Heartbeats*.

Epilogue
If Your Dream Stays a Dream

You might think that it is easy for me to be positive, especially at this time of my life. Afterall, I got rid of my bleedings and my IVF was successful with the end result being that I birthed two precious, wonderful children. I am beyond grateful that I got blessed with my babies and that my suffering from hemorrhaging and bleedings has finally been lifted. The price I paid, in my emotional, mental, and physical wellbeing was high, but I remain full of gratitude.

My deepest wish is that everyone that wants to get rid of their chronic physical challenges like PCOS, endo, or cysts, has their wish come to fruition. I also deeply wish that those of you longing for a child have their wish come true.

However, as painful as it is to say, not all wishes come true and not all dreams are fulfilled. If this is where you have landed, and if this has become your reality, you have my deepest care, empathy and longest of hugs. This is where it becomes really hard and a heavy burden to carry.

If you have come to the end of the IVF journey and there is no baby, you can feel crushed with your whole world and existence feeling unbearable. It is devastating and extremely difficult to absorb, let alone comprehend. I can't imagine how you are really feeling, but I think I got a small insight after my IVF miscarriage, and I will share how I felt to try to support you and your Trauma with a capital "T."

For many years, I felt robbed from not being able to get pregnant. For many years, I also felt robbed from not being able to give birth naturally and normally. I dreamed of having a baby where fertilization occurred after a natural act of love with my husband and having a birth that was peaceful and normal. But none of this happened. None of this was my destiny. After my miscarriage, I was devasted. I was hurting so deeply. I was lonely and felt empty. With that came so many feelings of grief, sadness, weariness, and hopelessness. I knew I had to allow myself to feel all of those feelings and to grieve to take some kind of step forward again at some point in time.

If you do not get what you dream of, I want you to know that it hurts. It hurts deep inside where you can feel empty. Allow yourself to feel those feelings and allow yourself to grieve. Even if you tried everything and did your best and ended up in a place you did not anticipate, you now need to allow yourself to fully feel and not stuff down any feelings. If you are in a place right now where you are not getting what you have been longing for, allow yourself to feel the emptiness within you. Allow yourself to find comfort in the darkness so that you can soon find the light.

Along the way, please remember that you have done all in your power to be successful, but for some mysterious reason(s), it did not work. You can feel small, shameful, not worthy, useless and many other feelings at this time. I did. I did many times. These feelings were all parts and pieces of the previous versions of myself and were also residing in my current self.

Again, I invite you to feel the feelings. Feelings are necessary. Feel them so you can release them, move on, and let go. It is different for everyone and takes different amounts of time. But I am here to tell you to feel all the feelings so you can move on to release them and somehow move forward. You did your best and it is not your fault. IT IS NOT YOUR FAULT. You are a wonderful person no matter what. Never forget that. Here is a beautiful way to think about healing your nervous system and feeling your feelings. It is from @healwithbritt on Instagram:

Your nervous system heals every time
you allow anger to be heard.
Your nervous system heals every time
you allow fear to be felt.
Your nervous system heals every time
you validate your tears.
Your nervous system heals every time
you lean into discomfort.
Your nervous system heals every time
you express instead of suppress.
Your nervous system heals when you reconnect
with its natural rhythm, its primal wisdom, and
its ancient release of feelings, emotions, and sensation.
~ LET YOURSELF HEAL ~

This takes time, so give yourself the gift of time. Also, allow yourself to access your feelings with grace. What is grace, you might ask? Grace is walking gently by your own side, being open-minded with yourself, and being kind and caring to yourself. Grace, for me, has played many roles. It has helped me to be kinder to myself, especially my inner self. It has allowed be to also be more aware of what my needs are, like I would be to a dear friend. You need time to forgive yourself through your own grace or kindness.

Your body is a miracle even if it does not work the way you

want. Scream out loud, hit pillows, go boxing, write down in a journal, and do whatever you need to do to let the hurting feelings out. When you let them out, the self-forgiveness can start. Forgive your body to be able to heal. Forgive your brain for feeding you obsessive thoughts. Forgive your heart for not loving yourself enough. Forgive family and friends for what they may or may not have done to help you, but instead hurt you. Try to focus on love and compassion instead. It might be and feel hard at this time, but little by little, step by step you can see all the great things about your body and life.

One way to help you heal and be able to see the good things in life and find self-love, compassion, and joy again is to fill your cup. What fills your cup? Write a list with all the things that might fill your cup, which really means, that which brings you joy. On my list are walking in nature, a bath, a good cup of coffee, talking to a friend, a massage, a nap in the middle of the day, dancing, singing, baking, and cuddling with my dog, to mention some. Get a paper and pen and write a list with everything that fills your cup. Add things as soon as you come up with a new idea. Next step is to do at least one thing on your list each day. Even if you don't feel like it, do at least one. Grab something from your list and enjoy. Action is distraction, and that is what you need now.

Another tool is walking through life with the attitude of gratitude. I mentioned that in this book and encourage you to think of or write down three things each day that you are grateful for or happy about. Start a gratitude journal. We tend to need five positive thoughts to eliminate one negative. Using this method to acknowledge good things in life helps you shift your mind and life. When you are in a state of gratitude, you cannot be in any other state of mind.

When you are ready, there are other ways to experience, feel and give love.

Shared Heartbeats

When my kids were ten years old, we got a puppy. That is my newest little baby, and my kids call him little brother. As I have shared, we can find love and share our love in many ways even if we would want it in one particular way. We can adopt, foster, get a puppy, or some other way to fill our lives with love, care, and joy.

I am also so grateful to have two godsons. One is an adult, and one is just a couple of years old. Even if we live with a continent between us, it brings me so much love and joy to be so connected to these humans as their godmother! What an honor! Today, we can Facetime and send videos so easily. I even play hide and seek on the phone! These two precious souls are a part of my life and help to fill my cup. I am hoping that you, too, have others like this in your life or will.

As I have mentioned, if you do not get your dream, take the critical time to feel and grieve.

Then, when you least expect it, you will find a new dream to feel and to share your love and joy within your life. You will find it, maybe not the way you think, but that is ok. Sometimes life surprises us and gives us something that is even better than what we were dreaming of or longing for. In the meantime, fill your heart with all the wonderful blessings life has to offer to you right now.

I'm sending you a big hug and promise you that one day, it <u>will</u> feel better. You will get to the other side of this. For now, wrap your arms around yourself and feel the hug, please.

Thank You

Thank **YOU** for reading my book! You took precious time out of your life to help yourself, and this is what truly makes me happy!

Thank You to my husband and my two "Mirakel" children, for supporting me every way possible, for loving me every way possible, and for making my heart and soul dance and sing.

Thank You to my mom and dad for all of your care and support. I love you. I look forward to the adventures yet to come as we continue doing life together. I also am sending love out to my brother.

A HUGE thank you to my Book and Life Coach Lisa Steele George! This has been so much fun with your expert guidance and insights. I healed as I wrote and I enjoyed all our times together. Forever in my heart.

Thank you to my advanced readers, Anna, Ina, Linda, Malin, and Liselott, for your time and input. It means a lot to me. You are awesome!

To my dear, lovely, and close friends in my sisterhood, you all know who you are! You are supportive, loving, and caring, and you make me laugh! Thank You, each and every one of you, for the person you are and what you mean to me.

Finally, thank you to myself, that I dared to become so vulnerable! That I dared to put myself out there! And, that I ultimately finished this project of a lifetime.

About the Author

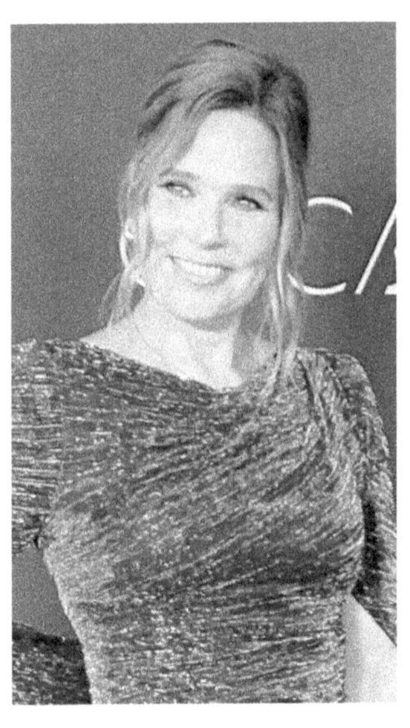

Annika Östberg was born and raised in South Sweden with her family. When her puberty started, she experienced major troubles with horrible, debilitating cramps, extended bleeding during menstruation, and chronic fatigue. These symptoms endured for twenty-five years before she was finally diagnosed with endometriosis. Annika battled through her heavy, long periods, horrible cramps, endometriosis, and cysts, and eventually went through IVF. She has tremendous experience with many different doctors and treatments in several countries. It took many years, a lot of struggles, pain, tears, and a fight to be in the healthy place she is today.

Annika knows how hard it is to not be taken seriously by others, including the medical community, when experiencing these kinds of pains. She also knows how much you have to fight to receive the help you need and how much healing has to occur along the way to teach yourself how not to be made to feel stupid, bad, or ashamed for the shortcomings of your body. Annika has experienced a lot during this journey and learned through curiosity, an innate longing to dig deep for knowledge, and a drive to understand her body, mind, and spirit.

Annika has moved a lot and lived in many different countries. She is fluent in Swedish, English, and German. Her diploma in Child and Youth Training and a master's degree in science and Math have served her well. She started as a teacher and currently is a certified Wellness Coach. During her life journey, Annika has also succeeded in becoming a certified Mindfulness and Pilates Instructor, a certified yoga instructor for kids and teens, an expert with food as medicine, a Reiki Master healer, a certified Crystal Singing Bowl healer, a diploma in Hawaiian Heart works Lomi Lomi massage and a diploma in Body and Life Success Training.

Annika is passionate about helping other people to feel their best inside out and help them heal them from their suffering. Annika is a Highly Sensitive Person (HSP) person and empath. She has learned to use the superpowers these personality traits give her to better understand other people, her space, and situations. She loves to spend time in nature and with her family, friends, and her beautiful dog, Piff. Singing, painting, dancing, baking, cooking, and exercising are things that make her life more beautiful.

Annika loves to make other people feel great, laugh, and have a good time. She is in the middle of her "second spring" as referred to by Chinese medicine during a woman's time of menopause. She is gaining the deeper knowledge needed about hormones and harmony for this time in her life. She is not a member of the Swedish House Mafia (music group), but Annika is a proud Swedish House Witch and enjoys working in her mysterious ways!

Above all else, Annika wants her readers to enjoy the ride of reading and experiencing this book and the insights, knowledge, and hope that you will receive! you!

To find out more about her, what she does, and her services, please check out her home page at this link: Healthbalance-joy.one

Appendix A

PERSONAL DIARY CONTENT: EVIL ENDO &
LAPORASCOPY DETAILS

(Feel free to enjoy reading this extra content taken directly from
my personal diary.)

There is an evil aspect to endometriosis that I must share with you, as it was one that I never considered nor did I expect. Endo can make its return to you after you are pregnant and after you have given birth. Endo does not necessarily go away, disappear, or even subside after a pregnancy or birth. In fact, the opposite happened to me. The severity of endometriosis after I was pregnant and after I gave birth was the worst ever, as it returned with a vengeance.

This came as a complete shock to me, my husband and even my ob-gyn. And, once again, the lack of awareness to this possibility still shocks me, as does the lack of my medical team (including IVF team) not informing me of this possibility.

The longer a woman has it, the worse it gets too. Why was

none of this shared with me? Why wasn't I educated? This is astounding, ridiculous & outright shocking. It was actually a friend of mine that sent me a newspaper article (a real cut out paper, newspaper article) with a list of symptoms that cued me into the idea of endo for the first time. That was after I gave birth, when my symptoms flared up again. It took twenty-five years to diagnose my endometriosis, twenty-five years. My symptoms started at the tender age of fifteen, in the year of 1987. I was forty years old, in the year of 2012, when I was finally diagnosed, after I shared that article with my ob-gyn.

When I wrote this chapter, I took the time to reflect on all the surgeries I had as well along the endo journey. I had five in total, all that came after the pregnancy & birth.

Here they are:

1. C-section.
2. Abdomen surgery to remove scar tissue. Much worse pain than a c-section due to the cutting of so much tissue.
3. Removal of my uterus, due to endo. The twins were five years old at this time. I was advised to keep my tubes and my ovaries to avoid early menopause.
4. Cysts that were removed were attached to the stomach wall, ovary, and bowels. Both tubes had to be removed this time as well, due to scar tissues, and one ovary. Kept one ovary to avoid menopause. This was all due to the continued growth of endo scar tissues.
5. Kidney stone surgery to release the stones and to remove more scar tissue. After this, I could finally use the toilet as needed. It took a long time to heal.

CYSTS AND LAPAROSCOPY

I so remember the cyst situation in such detail, as if it was just yesterday. It started when I was in so much pain, after New Year's 2014, that I went to the emergency room. I had pain in the ovary on the right side and thought that there was a cyst there that did not want to break on its own. The pain had increased over a full week. I was afraid that it would continue, when my husband would be gone on a business trip and I would be alone with the children. Here is a list of the most common symptoms of cysts:

- Pelvic pain.
- Bloating.
- Pressure on your bladder making it feel like you have to urinate a lot.
- Painful menstruation.
- Pain during intercourse.
- Nausea and vomiting.

Immediately when I got to the hospital, I was put on a drip and then I went for an ultrasound, both on the stomach and vaginally. I asked what she saw, and she was not allowed to say. It is sent to the doctor for h/she to discuss it with me. Europe's process is a bit different from the US. In Europe, you can see on the screen while the technician is working. They will also share with you what they see directly. Then a CAT scan was done, and I really felt like I would pee on myself. They said that the cyst was not that worrying, but that there was too much scar tissue in my intestine, so it was probably scar tissue that had grown and was in the way. I had to go home and would try to make an appointment with my gynecologist within a day or two. If it got worse, I was instructed to come back. I had already called earlier and got an appointment for a gynecologist, but there was a waiting period, so now it was good that I had that time left. The appointment was for the coming week. My gynecologist was actually named Dr. Love or "The Love Dr." as I called him. Interesting name for the profession he has!

When I saw him, he immediately felt that there was a cyst. I felt much pain, too, when he felt it, and then he said that with the documents I had brought from the emergency room, he had to do an operation. If it felt better in a few days, I could have waited, but it would probably end with an operation anyway. My appointment was scheduled for the 13th of February. I was shaken when I went home from the reception. Not another surgery. It was barely over the year mark since the last operation. But he thought it had grown together and that it was, therefore, difficult to go to the bathroom and do number two. The cyst and ovary could also be involved.

LAPAROSCOPY DETAILS

We relocated to America Jan 2013, and what I am writing about happened in 2014, as described in short above. I was really in pain, horrible pain that radiated down my leg, and it felt like I had a hard tennis ball down right by one of my ovaries and above my groin. Simple yoga moves and soft posture were not pleasant at all.

When I was told that it was a month until the operation, I was not happy. It's maybe quite fast in some eyes, but I wanted to do it, and have it overdone because I hurt all the time. I could only sleep on my back. If I turned on my side, I was waking up from a stabbing in my stomach. I also had a pillow between my knees because it hurt to lie with my legs straight. I was a real romantic monster!

I started googling babysitters and nannies to prepare for help with the kids, but it was not so easy at short notice to find someone. I was so happy when I spoke to my mom on the phone. My parents said they could come and support when I had the laparoscopy surgery. It was such a relief to have such wonderful and healthy parents who could step up and support me at this time! We booked tickets, and they arrived from Sweden to the US the week before the surgery.

The week I was scheduled for surgery, my husband was in India, so it was great to have help with the children from a family that they and I knew. The Friday before the surgery, I took my mother to the day spa. I tried to relax but already had a headache in the morning and in the afternoon. It was a migraine with nausea, so I had to go to bed blindfolded. I was so nervous about this surgery. The weekend before my parents came, I was so worried and nervous because then I knew it was getting closer. This was the fourth operation in six years, and I knew a little about what I had to go through.

I had been instructed to shower with a special soap the night before and to sleep in a clean bed with clean pajamas. On the morning of the surgery, I would shower with the soap again and wash my hair. I was instructed to not use any kind of skin cream, deodorant, or makeup. I put on clothes that were easy to put on and take off and that didn't sit tight on my stomach. I wore tights and a dress with a cardigan. A friend picked me and my mother up after we had left the children at preschool and drove us to the hospital. When we're more than halfway there, I check to make sure I have my phone with me, and of course, it's gone. We turn around and I run in and look, and my dad says you put it in the bag. I had put flip flops on, an apple, newspaper, etc., so it was quite full in the bag, and when I turned it upside down, the phone fell into my hands. So back again and we were a little late.

I was supposed to be at the hospital at nine-thirty, but we were probably ten minutes late. But it didn't seem to do anything.

We were enrolled. I already had a bracelet on my wrist since I took a blood test two days earlier. Since the night before, I hadn't eaten anything, and my stomach grumbled a bit. I was brought into a small booth with a bed and appliances, and they told me to take off all my clothes, put them in a blue bag, and pull for a curtain. On the bed was a "dress" with an open back and a couple of strings to tie with. It looks the same everywhere in the world, I think, and they all are a bit boring, beige color that seems to be the worldwide color. There are similar ones in both Sweden and Germany. I had to go pee in a jar and then go to bed. They came and measured blood pressure, fever, etc., and a nurse put a drip in the left hand. Then she said that for this operation, they wanted one in each arm.

When she tried to put an IV in my right hand, it was not so easy. Apparently, I have small vessels and they wanted a certain size of needle. What was new was that I got a small burning sting first so it wouldn't feel so much when they drove into the vein. I had worried about that moment because it hurt so much last time. On the third attempt, she succeeded and that time with a smaller size of the needle. A week and a half later, there was still a large blue-green patch on my forearm!

When everything was rigged, they called Mom in. We waited a while, and then the doctor came. He said he would take a good look and check everything. If both ovaries were bad, he would take both, and if that was the case, I would get some device so I didn't end up in menopause right away. So, if there were a device plugged in when I woke up, I would know.

It felt good to talk to him, and I said that he had to do what was needed and that I would rather not end up in this situation again soon. Then some nurses and a PhD student came and said now you get something that makes you relax. Like a glass of wine, I thought! Well, more like a whole bottle was the answer. We rolled a few meters away, and I waved goodbye to a Mom, who walked out the doors to the waiting room, we didn't even make it another two meters before I passed out and don't remember anything.

There was a robot used for my laparoscopy surgery. There were four entry points made for four incision points through my body. One incision was in through my belly button. When they finally did get to the cyst, **they found the tennis ball-sized cyst that connected itself to many things in my body: my right ovary, my stomach wall, and my bowels.** I've bolded this and italicized it because it needs to stand out in my diary and really scream out: ENDO IS EVIL! Can you even imagine? I could not when they told me. No wonder I was in such pain. No wonder I felt like complete crap while not being able to even take a successful crap!

I woke up, and someone asked how I was doing. I feel that it hurts a lot in the lower right side of my stomach. I say that and that I'm terribly cold. I get something through the needle, and it feels good. The person also asks if I want to see Mom, but I feel so bad and have a hard time opening my eyes. I don't want her to see me like that, so I say they can wait. I also get a quilt that blows hot air into it. nice. The next time I woke up, it felt better.

The person asks again if mom should come in, and I say it's probably best. She must be worried, I think. Before mother comes in, the man removes the tube in my nose and lots of electrodes on my chest. He asks if I want to be more roasted or toasted and I answer that it's nice. The warm air blanket may remain. Mom comes in, and she's worried. When she sees me, she anxiously wonders how it is and if I have a fever. She got to talk to the doctor at one o'clock. She would talk and talk, as much as she could understand what he told her. She knows English, but not that much.

I remember that I didn't want to wake up after the anesthesia.

I talked to her a little, but it's exhausting and hurts my throat. It's hard to keep your eyes open. After an hour, a nurse comes and says that I can stay overnight as I am so weak and in pain. When she takes off the warm air blanket, she finds a large ice pack where the ice has melted. No wonder you froze, she says cheerfully. I am rolled up in a hallway. There is another woman in the room behind a curtain. Mom is already there. She was not allowed to go the same way that I did. We call my friend, who comes to pick up Mom at seven. I am thirsty and get something that looks like a lollipop but is a stick with a piece of foam rubber on it that is dipped in water and moisturizes the lips. Better than nothing.

I thought I would get something small to eat, but no. I doze off and wake up when they come and check my blood pressure, fever, etc. The night staff comes, and I say it hurts again. When I see her preparing a syringe, I think no, not another syringe. But she puts it in the drop. Geez, it's starting to burn in the wrist. I say that, and she stops and injects more slowly. The night nurse introduces himself, and his name is Nils. I say it sounds Swedish, and he says his grandfather is from Sweden.

He's a funny guy and tells my roommate that she shouldn't be sad when soon he and I are going to go up and have a dance to the toilet. At eleven, we try to go to the toilet. I don't need to pee at all, but I must try, says Nils. It hurts to get up. I'm dizzy and can only take small steps. But in the few meters to the toilet, I hold on to the drop stick with one hand while Nils holds on tight to my other arm. I walk backward to the toilet and Nils helps me hold up the dress and holds me when I try to sit down.

I also hold tightly to the handle on the wall and manage to sit down. I was trying to pee, and to my surprise, a small stream came out. Nils stands outside and tells me to tell him when I'm done. I sit for a long time, and a little comes all the time. After all that energy exerted, I thought for sure that the whole toilet bowl would be full! They had inserted a measurement bowl into the toilet to check my output. But as they put it in to measure how much I did, it was really little. It also felt like I was dipping my butt into it as well! When it's over, I call out to Nils in my weak voice. When I have called three times, and no one comes, I pull the string. In one second, he's coming. I have toilet paper in my hand but can't get myself up from the toilet or turn around to wipe my ass off! How embarrassing!

So, when he holds my arm, I wipe my ass, and then we slowly go back to my bed. So nice to have a hospital bed where the back section goes up with pressing a button and when I've got my legs up, I can just lean back and slowly go down to lying down with this button! The night's sleep time includes many interruptions when the staff comes. It also included times when my roommate vomits. I remember how early in the mornings the nurses would come and wake us up, always before six o'clock, to come and do the morning medical checks.

I don't understand why I should call the kitchen by myself to order breakfast. I have received a small brochure and what I can choose from is tea, coffee, lemon sorbet, jelly or so. I asked a nurse how to order at half past eight, when I'm hungry, and my roommate has had breakfast. Another nurse comes in and shares with me that she was at the surgery yesterday and wants to check on me as my doctor can't. She says the operation went well and hopes I will feel better soon. She says that I should eat a real breakfast. I'm so happy! It was last Wednesday night that I ate, now it's Friday morning, and the smell of coffee is wonderful. She gives me a new menu with much more to choose from. So, I check the new menu and order coffee, apple juice, natural yogurt, fresh fruit bowl and goes on with scrambled eggs and bacon.

My breakfast time feels luxurious! I carefully sip the juice to check that it doesn't make me nauseous. It's going well and I eat everything. I ask when I can go home, and they say I have to get up and go for a walk first. My friend who can pick me up can only pick up until 11 am so I would like to be discharged by then. I go for a round with a nurse. It's fine with my drip stick to hold on to. I feel a little dizzy, but I don't say it. It's almost two hours before I ask again if I can go home soon. They tell me to go one more turn and I do. I say it's going well. (but honestly, it feels like crap, I am a little dizzy and my legs are week, but you choose your words). I really want to be picked up by my friend when she can. There is no cab in this area to call so I am depending on my friends.

WOMAN MADE OF STEEL

My roommate had similar surgery as I had. When talking to her a little bit one morning, she shared with me that she was wondering what kind of woman I am, because "obviously I was made of steel." She goes on to talk about when the nurses ask how much pain we have, you must answer on a scale from one to ten, where ten is being hit by a car. She has answered seven or eight each time and I have answered two or three. I share with her that I compare this pain to the previous surgeries I have had, and that I imagine being hit by a car equates to having pain at the ten level. A nurse comes and removes the drip and has a prescription for two painkillers and I get a painkiller so I can make it home. I got another painkiller shot in the drip in the morning, but she thinks I need some more before the trip home and I'm not saying no.

She tells me that they ordered a wheelchair to take me down to the entrance. A handsome older gentleman in a red jacket and tie comes and drives me down to the entrance and waits with me until my friend arrives and he drives me out to the car. The trip home is going well even though it is bumpy, as the roads are so potholed after the severe winter. It hurts quite a lot. I come home and my parents help me to bed. Difficult to lie down when you don't have the good folding backrest of a hospital bed! I get help from my dad and my husband, who arrives home this afternoon when I have to get up. When I need to get up and down, I have to put my hands around their necks, and they grab my back and pull me up. It feels as if everything in the stomach is being moved around and rearranged and it hurts.

It hurts so bad that I get dizzy and must sit on the edge of the bed for a while before I can get help standing up. I sleep reasonably well at night with the heating pad in the back and two pillows under the knees. I wake up and feeling okay on Saturday morning. Magnus brings breakfast in bed. He helps me sit up, and I eat a small yogurt and a toasted sandwich and drink coffee. I'm in a bit of pain and take one of the pain pills that Magnus brought from the pharmacy. Then I read a magazine. Suddenly, I start to feel sick. I call for help to lie down, but no one hears my weak voice. After shouting a few times, I take a medicine can and throw it at the wall. Then I throw another one. It is painful just to throw the small can. Then my son hears something knocking and comes to ask what it says. I tell him to call dad.

Magnus comes and helps me into bed. Mom also comes and puts pillows under my legs so they come up high. I'm dizzy and terribly ill and say I can't get to the toilet, so they have to get a bucket. I really don't want to puke! Just the thought of having to use my ripped stomach for that is horrible. Then I lie there all morning feeling sick and faint. Strange that you can feel so faint when you are lying down. My skin crawls and feels strange, and I think, lucky I get to die at home, I thought. It felt so miserable. Dam, I was feeling so bad!

At lunch, I manage, with help, to get to the kitchen and eat some potato and carrot soup that my mother made, and then I lie down and feel miserable again all afternoon. In the evening, I eat some fish and potatoes and then lie on the sofa. We're going to check out the Eurovision Song Contest from Europe on television. But I don't see much of it. I must close my eyes so I don't feel too bad. Magnus gives me a salty candy that I love. I lick it a little gently and it's enough to make me almost throw up. No more candy for me tonight!

I wake up feeling pretty good and roll out of bed on. My stomach hurts a bit but it's not as bad as the days before. I actually feel good enough to get up and start making breakfast for my children and parents. I cannot carry the heavier stuff like milk and juice packs to the table, but my strong, healthy son does. I am completely exhausted after breakfast and using the toilet, and in pain after this excursion. I take a painkiller and doze off in bed.

Today's other big thing is that I take a walk to the mailbox (20 meters) and am outside for a little while. After some freshly baked chocolate cake, I'm back in bed dozing off. After an hour I think now it's time and pull myself up to sit in bed and pick up the computer and write down the beginning of this. Magnus is with grandma and the children at swimming school, but soon they will be home. Now I'm going to help grandpa heat up the wok leftovers from last week until they arrive. What an eventful day. And it's not over yet!

It took several weeks before I could move reasonably normally. Simple things hurt, like pushing a cart in the store or lifting things, for example. It took over a year before it felt like most of it was healed but I can feel all the scar tissue. It hurts when it passes through the gut sometimes and I must hold on to something and breathe deeply to cope with the pain. It passes quite quick so the pain does not last for long but it is like someone stab you with a knife or something sharp.

Appendix B

EXERCISES AND TOOLS FOR SUPPORTING YOUR
WELLBEING

Morning Rituals

These can be done anytime in your day/evening but are wonderful for your mornings.

Angel Wings

Stand with your legs hip wide apart. Have a little bend in your knees and feel that you have a straight, tall posture. With an inhale through your nose, raise both your arms straight above your head. Hold your breath shortly when your reach up to the sky. As you slowly exhale through your mouth, let your arms come down to your side.

Side Stretch

Reach up your arms above your head as you inhale and with an exhale, lean to one side. Feel a nice stretch on your side and how it stretches a bit more with your inhale. After a few breaths on an inhale, come back to a straight up position and with nest exhale lean to the other side and feel the nice stretch on that side for a few breaths. With an inhale come to center and with an exhale slowly let your arms sinks down to your sides.

Shoulder Roll

Roll your shoulders up to your ears then back, down and to the front before your roll up again. Add your breathing. When you roll up and back, you inhale and down and to the front you exhale. This is a slow, gentle movement that loosen up your tight shoulders. If it feels good switch direction after a while.

Knocking on Heaven's Door

Put your feet and legs a little bit wider with toes facing out. Try to hold the lower part of your body still as you gentle swing your heavy loose arms from side to side. Let your arms gentle hit your body like a soft massage. Check that your shoulders and jar are relaxed.

The Rag Doll

Bend down and let your full palms or just fingers touch the floor. Bend your knees if you need. With both palms and feet on the ground, take some deep breaths and feel how you fill up the space between your ribs in your back. After a few breaths, lift up your hands and let them hand down. Your head hangs loose and your jaw is relaxed. If it feels good, rock from side to side. With a good bend in your knees, you slowly roll all the way up to a standing position.

Sit On a Chair

Stand with your legs hip wide apart. Tighten your core and with an inhale you reach your arms in front of you at the same time as you sit down on an imaging chair. As you rise up to a standing position, squeeze your glutes together and feel how your shoulder blades move closer to each other in the back. Sit down on the "chair" ten times.

Shake Off

Shake off your body for a moment! Shake your hands and legs and feel how your let go of tensions and get new energy! You have done some exercises and stretches and are ready to go out and face the day. Enjoy your day!

Exercises for Anytime

Breathing Minute

For this exercise, you can stand up or sit down. If it feels all right, close your eyes for better focus. Take a deep inhale through your nose, filling up your lungs all the way down to your belly. Fill your belly up with air like it is a balloon. Hold your breath and then slowly exhale through your mouth. In yoga, we often say, fill up on ease, exhale out stress. If you like, put a timer on one minute, but you can normally do three to four breaths this way for one minute. Feel how the slow breathing calms down your system and gives you newer energy. This will also help you concentrate better, get better sleep and focus. Do it several times during your day to help your body slow down and recharge.

Energy Hook Up and Balance

Start with soft tapping on your cheeks. That is where acupressure points starts and you activate them. Then move down to tap just under your collarbone. After some tapping there move down between your breast and tap the thymus. After that, you tap your sides a bit under your armpits. That is spleen and your support to digest food and thoughts. This little exercise starts your meridians and lymphatic system and gives you energy, balance, and calm at the same time.

Grounding

You can do grounding in many ways. Here is one way of doing it. Start with sitting in a position that suits you like on a chair, with a straight back, and your feet on the ground. Allow your eyes to close and take some deep breaths in through your nose and out of your mouth. Let your shoulder sink down. Feel your feet on the floor. In your imagination, see how your meridians lengthen and grow longer and down in the ground. They spread in all directions, and you feel stable. At the same time, you feel how your meridians grow tall and above your head. Reaching high up in all directions, you are now connected with heaven and earth. Feel a light from above slowly go down your head, spine, and legs and down to your feet and ground. The light updates and upgrades every cell, tissue, muscle, and your DNA. You feel refreshed. From the ground, a spiral-twists up, around your whole body and connects with the sky. It forms a bubble or balloon with six feet around your body. You feel safe and protected. You are now grounded, connected, protected, and supported. Take a deep breath in and then exhale, and slowly open your eyes.

Body Points to Hold to Give Support During Your Period

Front Head

Just hold your full palm sidelong on your front head for a while. You can touch your front head or just hover above. Close your eyes and feel the energy. Or ask a friend to hold their hand on your front head.

Rooster

Put your palms together in front of you. Then, move them so one palm starts at your front head and fingers go up your head and the other hand the palm is in your neck and finger go up your head. Hold for a little time and feel the energy. These two hand holdings support acupressure points that support and balance your female genitals.

Self-Massage to Support Your Lymphatic System.

This could be a great exercise when you take a shower, but you can do it dry to or when your put on a body lotion. If you are in the shower and just took some soap you start at your feet massaging up your legs. Then move to your hand and massage up your arm. Then the other arm. Massage gentle and a bit more around your armpits since there are more lymphatic nots to activate. Massage your face and down to your neck and hold your hands with fingers pressed in a bit on the back of your neck and slowly pull forward and massage with your fingertips from your shoulder down your collarbone like rain drops. Massage around your bellybutton with both hands and then pull up along your sides to your armpits. Shake off your arms and legs.

YouTube Meditations

Search for Children's Mindfulness Meditation. Some of my favorites are "My Treehouse" or The Fairy Garden." They are about fifteen minutes long and help you relax, feel renewed, filled with love, joy and so much more satisfied over all. Kids" stuff is sometimes the best!

Detox for Gut Support

Keeping your body running clean and efficiently is important. It helps to keep regular bowel movements, clean out old stuff, and to get rid of bacteria and viruses that may be harboring in your system(s). Hence, a detox is helpful. I recommend that you start your morning with a glass of orange juice or water and add one tablespoon of Psyllium Husk, let it sit for a couple of minutes and then drink or eat like Jell-O. There are so many natural benefits to Psyllium Husk. It is a natural type of fiber that acts as a gentle laxative and just to keep things moving regularly. It helps to manage blood levels as well as for heart health. Try to drink plenty of water to support the detox. Do this for 3-5 days, and then maybe once a month or every second week till you feel better and your bowels move better. You can get some gas from the bacteria and toxic stuff leaving the bowels, so just be aware of that and that it is normal.

Another great way to start your day is to add a splash of apple cider vinegar or fresh squeezed lemon and drink this in a glass of lukewarm water the first thing in the morning. That supports your body with gentle cleaning and to avoid glucose spikes.

Another way to support your wellbeing is to eat on a regular basis. Try to eat breakfast, lunch, and dinner at the same time most of your days, with dinner preferably around 6pm. If you need to, you can have a morning or afternoon snack, but please try to select a snack that supports you like fruit, nuts, seeds, carrots, or other veggies. Veggies are great with some hummus or guacamole.

If you would like to try a meal plan, you can find one at my home page: www.Healthybalancejoy.one

Your Support People

In chapter 8, Partner Relationship and Pillar People, I talk a lot about finding your support people, the ones you can trust to be part of your inner circle for guidance, love, and support. Maybe some of the doctors and professionals that provide the above services become part of this network for you! At first, you may not feel this way. But eventually, you will know which ones nestle their way into your heart. They will be the ones you respect, trust, and become your partners in your struggles to get pregnant. They become part of your intimate journey, are sympathetic ears for listening to your stories as well as sharing stories with you of other women who have fought and survived the same battles. Enjoy these humans. Embrace their truth and allow yourself to become a believer.

Resources

In this book, most content is from my own personal life experiences, but I did receive a lot of knowledge and motivation from many inspirational people and teachers in my life that I want to acknowledge. First of all, I am so grateful for all the wonderful people that have come into my life to share their knowledge, wisdom, and ways to heal. I cannot even begin to know where we would be in this world without our educators and healers.

Second, the following is a list of the most important people/resources I learned from in one way or another, and who have influenced me, in no particular order:

- Tina Göransson and Annelie Nyqvist's book called *The Key to Health* and her Moxa workshop in Hermansdal, Sweden. A great workshop.
- *Happy Bodies Studio* by Maria, a Swedish yoga instructor with a studio in Sweden with wonderful workshops, including *Body and Life Success*. I am a graduate of this workshop!

- Ifigenia Psari, at *Life Direction*, Wellbeing and Holistic Coach in Sweden whom I have worked with for many years. She has been instrumental in helping me get off some meds.
- Dr. Diamantis, specializes in Chinese medicine. His books *Hormonell Harmoni, Den Holistiska Vagen* and *Key to Your Health* are excellent! His workshops are as well.
- Maria Borelius, a science journalist, health coach and author of, *Health Revolution* and *Bliss*. Great reads.
- Kay Pollack, author, film maker and provides workshops which inspired me so much! He is a wonderful teacher and educator. His movies are also wonderful.
- Agneta Sjödin, author of *A Woman's Journey* and *From Your Own Power* and her Swedish podcast called *Into Your Soul*. I've read these books and recommend them.
- Kristin Kaspersen and her books called *Good Food, Good Morning,* and *Thankfulness*. Take a listen to and enjoy her podcast.
- Susanne Jönsson, a Swedish teacher and coach at Helhetscentrum, and her books.
- Anette Kozica, a Swedish health coach at Mistelgården. She offers life changing retreats, ones that helped me turn my life around.
- Carina and Janne, spiritual artist, and a cranial sacral/lymphatic healer with their wonderful B&B in south Sweden called Ängshyddan. They are angels on this earth who helped me through many rough years.
- Jenny Åsenlund, a Swedish Professional Coach and Yoga Instructor with wonderful retreats and

workshops around *Soulful Entrepreneur*. Jenny is a wonderful friend.

- Donna Lakes, founder, owner and teacher at Ascension Healing Art School, Ferndale, Michigan, USA. She has become one of my friends. I enjoy helping out at her Center as an energy and reiki teacher, along with inner child healing. I received my Reiki Master and Inner Child Healing education certificates here!
- Donna Eden offers workshops and books on energy medicine. My learnings around energy medicine originated here.
- Joe Dispenza, a US author and who offers motivating workshops, and most famous book *"Becoming Supernatural"* and *Breaking the Habit of Being Yourself*.
- Louise Hay, internationally well-known author, and speaker. *The Power is Within You, Heal Your Body, You Can Heal Your Life* and *How to Love Yourself* will blow your mind!
- Bruce Lipton (author that focuses on the body with its natural powers), Andreas Goldemann (specialty is holistic focus, spirituality, and sound healing) and Mate Gabor (specialty is trauma) workshops. All of their books are excellent as well as their workshops. I have been blessed to attend many of these great healer's workshops.
- Dr. Ola Schenström at Mindfulness Center in Sweden. I received my mindfulness coaching certification from here.
- Angelica Henriksson and Josefin Wikström at Barnyoga.com with yoga for kids and teens with

trauma yoga for physical health. I received my yoga certifications from here.

- Johannes Cullberg, health coach in Sweden whom I highly recommend.
- Charlotta Rexmark, a Swedish spiritual wellness coach located in Sweden.
- Sonja Blessing, a German owner of *Heart Lomi Lomi Blessing.* I have been trained by her and have my certification for her Hawaiian Heart Lomi Lomi massage.
- Daniela Bärthlein, located in Germany. She is a Shiatsu and holistic coach who is also my guru who has taught and helped me a lot over many years.
- Eva Berlander, a Swedish author who also offers workshops. *To Live and Just Not Survive* and *You Can Make It Happen.* My husband and I fully experienced and enjoyed her "Live and Not Just Survive" workshop!
- Micke Gunnarsson, a Swedish entrepreneur, and coach.
- Anna Hallen, a Swedish health coach. I have read several books by her and recommend them.
- Malin Sandell Berggrensson and Ina Elverljung, retreats, and workshops for HSP (highly sensitive persons) I loved this retreat in Sweden!
- Rose Wisniewski, a Craniosacral Health and Wellness Coach, USA.
- Martina Carl, practices in Germany with a specialty in Physiotherapy. It is called "Heilkunde" in German. She has wonderful yoga classes.
- Kurt Rotter located in Germany. Owner and teacher at Body Balance Pilates. This is where I received my Pilates training and certifications.

- Hannah Teutscher, a former well-known ballet performer and owner of *Performance Fit Pilates* in Germany, but from the USA. I became close friends with her. She helped me a lot after my surgeries. She runs this amazing Pilates studio now with her husband.
- Dr. Klaus Just, ob-gyn, and his wife Sonja Just, who is a midwife (Hebamme, in German). They are located in Germany. She performed reiki on me which is how we discovered my blockages. She was also my caring and supportive midwife.
- Dana Fischer, owner of Pilates Method located in Birmingham, Michigan USA. This is where I currently practice Pilates on reformer.
- Jesse Inchauspe, NYT best seller author known as "The Glucose Goddess" who wrote *The Glucose Goddess Method.*
- Frida Tronnberg, owner of the company Helt Underliv, a pelvic floor health and education center. I learned a lot from her through her programs.
- Lisa Kock, a Swedish born Costa Rican shaman healer and holistic nature teacher, provides five-week workshops called: Heal with Nature. Highly recommended!
- Many dear friends, no one forgotten.
- My family, immediate and extended.

I have done so much research online and have read several studies about women's reproductive health and issues by Sahlgrenska Universitetssjukhuset, Carlanderska Sjukhuset, Kinderwunchcentrum in Nuernberg and learned from their studies online.

I have also been a Wellness Coach to many clients around

the world. I am still a Wellness Coach today. You can see that my back ground is wide, vast, and thorough. All of this **knowledge, which is power,** has been critical to my successful journey. I will continue coaching and helping clients by being in service to them and their conscious evolutions.

Notes

Notes

www.ingramcontent.com/pod-product-compliance
Lightning Source LLC
Chambersburg PA
CBHW060914140726
47996CB00001B/246